Physiotherapy in
OBSTETRICS

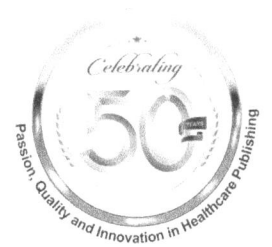

Physiotherapy in
OBSTETRICS

Namrata Kundariya MPT
Lecturer
Akar College of Physiotherapy
Ahmedabad, Gujarat India

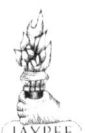

JAYPEE BROTHERS MEDICAL PUBLISHERS
The Health Sciences Publisher
New Delhi | London

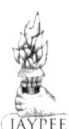 **Jaypee Brothers Medical Publishers (P) Ltd**

Headquarters
Jaypee Brothers Medical Publishers (P) Ltd
4838/24, Ansari Road, Daryaganj
New Delhi 110 002, India
Phone: +91-11-43574357
Fax: +91-11-43574314
Email: jaypee@jaypeebrothers.com

Overseas Office
J.P. Medical Ltd
83 Victoria Street, London
SW1H 0HW (UK)
Phone: +44 20 3170 8910
Fax: +44 (0)20 3008 6180
Email: info@jpmedpub.com

Website: www.jaypeebrothers.com
Website: www.jaypeedigital.com

© 2020, Jaypee Brothers Medical Publishers

The views and opinions expressed in this book are solely those of the original contributor(s)/author(s) and do not necessarily represent those of editor(s) of the book.

All rights reserved. No part of this publication may be reproduced, stored or transmitted in any form or by any means, electronic, mechanical, photocopying, recording or otherwise, without the prior permission in writing of the publishers.

All brand names and product names used in this book are trade names, service marks, trademarks or registered trademarks of their respective owners. The publisher is not associated with any product or vendor mentioned in this book.

Medical knowledge and practice change constantly. This book is designed to provide accurate, authoritative information about the subject matter in question. However, readers are advised to check the most current information available on procedures included and check information from the manufacturer of each product to be administered, to verify the recommended dose, formula, method and duration of administration, adverse effects and contraindications. It is the responsibility of the practitioner to take all appropriate safety precautions. Neither the publisher nor the author(s)/editor(s) assume any liability for any injury and/or damage to persons or property arising from or related to use of material in this book.

This book is sold on the understanding that the publisher is not engaged in providing professional medical services. If such advice or services are required, the services of a competent medical professional should be sought.

Every effort has been made where necessary to contact holders of copyright to obtain permission to reproduce copyright material. If any have been inadvertently overlooked, the publisher will be pleased to make the necessary arrangements at the first opportunity. The **CD/DVD-ROM** (if any) provided in the sealed envelope with this book is complimentary and free of cost. **Not meant for sale.**

Inquiries for bulk sales may be solicited at: jaypee@jaypeebrothers.com

Physiotherapy in Obstetrics

First Edition: **2020**

ISBN: 978-93-89188-66-0

Dedicated to

*My Father Mr Ravji Kundariya
and
My Mother Mrs Gita Kundariya
As always… their love, support and guidance
helped me to complete this project.*

Preface

This book is a study guide and reference for the physiotherapy students and clinicians practicing in the field of obstetrics. Obstetrics Physiotherapy has very wide scope in the field of physiotherapy. But we don't have much physiotherapy books for the students and practicing clinicians. I hope therapists and students will find this book useful and easy-to-use guide. The aim of writing this book is to provide systematic approach in assessing and treating obstetric patients and also preventing some obstetrics problems. This book will also be helpful to the physiotherapy students. This book covers most of the syllabus of well known universities like Gujarat University, Saurastra University, RK University, Rajiv Gandhi University, etc. Students will get all the necessary information from one book in easy to understand way.

The first chapter contains all the basics of obstetric anatomy and physiology. It contains all the necessary information required to understand obstetric physiotherapy.

Second chapter is all about the maternal biomechanics. Understanding biomechanics is very important for all the physiotherapists. By understanding biomechanics therapist will clearly understand the problems of pregnant women and also able to prevent and treat the problems of women during pregnancy.

Third chapter contains all details about antenatal and postnatal assessment of women. Fourth, fifth and sixth chapters cover the complete physiotherapy treatment and also the problems of pregnant women and its prevention during antenatal, postnatal and also during labor.

Seventh chapter covers the details about physiotherapy after cesarean section. Ninth chapter covers all the medical problems women may face during and after pregnancy. Eighth and tenth chapter is about the advanced techniques of painless labor and water birth.

Namrata Kundariya

Acknowledgments

I would like to thank my parents for their encouragement and helping me whenever I need. Their support played a large role in completion of this book.

I would like to thank Dr Priyanshu Rathod, Dean of School of Physiotherapy, RK University, Rajkot and Dr Meeta Patel (MD-Obstetrics and Gynecology) for their valuable guidance to improve this book.

I am also thankful to Mr Natvarlal Vasdadiya, artist of this book who helped me with all the illustrations and made this book easy-to-understand.

In the last my thanks go to Shri Jitendar P Vij (Group Chairman), Mr Ankit Vij (Managing Director), Mr MS Mani (Group President), Dr Madhu Choudhary (Publishing Head-Education), Ms Pooja Bhandari (Production Head), Ms Sunita Katla (Executive Assistant to Group Chairman and Publishing Manager), Ms Samina Khan (Executive Assistant to Publishing Head-Education), Ms Seema Dogra (Cover Visualizer), Mr Rajesh Sharma (Production Coordinator), Rajesh Ghurkundi (Graphic Designer), Deep Kumar (DTP Operator), Narsingh Kumar (Proof Reader) of M/s Jaypee Brothers Medical Publishers (P) Ltd, New Delhi, India, for giving me this opportunity.

Contents

CHAPTER 1: Maternal Anatomy and Physiology 1
- Female bony pelvis *1*
- Blood supply of the pelvic organs *3*
- Lymphatic drainage of the pelvis *6*
- Nerve supply of the pelvis *6*
- Changes in mammary glands during pregnancy *7*
- Hormonal control of ovulation *8*
- Female reproductive cycle *8*
- Anatomical and physiological changes during pregnancy *11*
- Pelvic floor muscles *17*

CHAPTER 2: Maternal Biomechanics 22
- Center of gravity *22*
- Changes in spine and pelvis *23*
- Posture *25*
- Gait *25*

CHAPTER 3: Approach to the Patient 28
- Diagnosis of pregnancy *28*
- Antenatal assessment *29*
- Postnatal assessment *38*

CHAPTER 4: Antenatal Physiotherapy 42
- Guidelines for exercise during pregnancy in healthy women *43*
- Contraindications to exercise during pregnancy *44*
- Benefits of exercise during pregnancy *45*
- Routine antenatal care *45*
- Exercise prescription *48*
- Antenatal physiotherapy for first trimester of pregnancy *48*
- Antenatal physiotherapy for second trimester of pregnancy *54*
- Antenatal physiotherapy for third trimester of pregnancy *61*
- Guidelines for managing the pregnant women *62*
- Sacroiliac joint pain/posterior pelvis pain/pelvic girdle pain *64*
- Effect of supine lying during pregnancy *65*

CHAPTER 5: Physiotherapy during Labor 69
- Stages of labor *69*
- Comfort measures to manage pain and suffering in labor *72*

CHAPTER 6: Postnatal Physiotherapy 84
- The effect of exercise on recovery from labor and delivery *85*
- Physiotherapy management guidelines *85*
- Ergonomic principles *86*
- Postural exercises *87*
- Immediate postnatal problems *88*
- Long-term postnatal problems *98*
- Abdominal muscle exercises *99*
- Training of pelvic movements *100*
- Pelvic floor awareness, training and strengthening *100*
- Warning signs to slow down *102*
- Advice on activities related to baby *102*
- General postnatal physiotherapy management protocol *103*

CHAPTER 7: Physiotherapy after Cesarean Section 108
- Indications of cesarean section *108*
- Postoperative physiotherapy management *109*
- Body mechanics *113*

CHAPTER 8: Painless Labor 115
- Epidural anesthesia *115*

CHAPTER 9: Common Medical Problems in Pregnancy 117
- Iron deficiency anemia *117*
- Pregnancy-induced hypertension or pre-eclampsia *118*
- Eclampsia *119*
- Polyhydramnios *119*
- Premature rupture of membrane *120*
- Intrauterine fetal death *120*
- Gestational diabetes mellitus (GDM) *120*
- Physiotherapy management *122*

Chapter 10: Water Birth 125
- Benefits of water birth *125*
- Risks of water birth *126*
- Contraindications for water birth *126*
    - *Glossary 127*
    - *Index 131*

Abbreviations

AIDS – **A**cquired **I**mmunodeficiency **S**yndrome

BMI – **B**ody **M**ass **I**ndex

BOS – **B**ase **O**f **S**upport

BP – **B**lood **P**ressure

COG – **C**enter **O**f **G**ravity

CS – **C**esarean **S**ection

EDD – **E**xpected **D**ate of **D**elivery

FSH – **F**ollicle **S**timulating **H**ormone

GDM – **G**estational **D**iabetes **M**ellitus

HIV – **H**uman **I**mmunodeficiency **V**irus

IVF – **I**n **V**itro **F**ertilization

LH – **L**uteinizing **H**ormone

LNMP – First day of the **L**ast **N**ormal **M**enstrual **P**eriod

MRI – **M**agnetic **R**esonance **I**maging

MTP – **M**edical **T**ermination of **P**regnancy

PGP – **P**elvic **G**irdle **P**ain

PIH – **P**regnancy-**I**nduced **H**ypertension

ROM – **R**ange **O**f **M**otion

SI Joint – **S**acro-**i**liac Joint

STD – **S**exually **T**ransmitted **D**isease

TENS – **T**ranscutaneous **E**lectrical **N**erve **S**timulation

TT – **T**etanus **T**oxoid

CHAPTER 1

Maternal Anatomy and Physiology

Chapter Outline
- Female Bony Pelvis
- Blood Supply of Pelvic Organs
- Lymphatic Drainage of Pelvis
- Nerve Supply of the Pelvic
- Changes in Mammary Glands during Pregnancy
- Hormonal Control of Ovulation
- Female Reproductive Cycle
- Anatomical and Physiological Changes during Pregnancy
- Pelvic Floor Muscles

INTRODUCTION

All living things reproduce. Reproduction is the process to continue species. The female reproductive system is divided into two groups: Internal and external. The internal genital organs are situated within the pelvis and it includes one pair that means two ovary and fallopian tubes, the single uterus and vagina. The external genital structures are collectively known as vulva and consist of mons pubis, pair of labia majora and minora single clitoris, vestibule of vagina and greater vestibular glands. Egg cells are also known as ova. Ovaries produce ova. After being produced, ova will go to uterus through fallopian tubes. Ova will become embryo and from embryo to fetus in the uterus.[1,2]

FEMALE BONY PELVIS

The articulated female pelvis comprises four bones: The two innominate bones, the sacrum and the coccyx. There are four joints in the pelvis namely the two sacroiliac joints, the pubic symphysis and the sacrococcygeal joint (Fig. 1.1). The pelvis is divided into two parts, the false pelvis (also known as pelvis major or greater pelvis) lying above the pelvic brim and the true pelvis (also known as pelvis minor or lesser pelvis) lying below the pelvic brim (Fig. 1.2).

False Pelvis[3]

False pelvis is also known as greater pelvis. Pelvic inlet is at the false pelvis. It is formed by iliac portion of innominate bones and limited above by iliac crests. Its obstetric function is to support enlarged uterus during pregnancy.

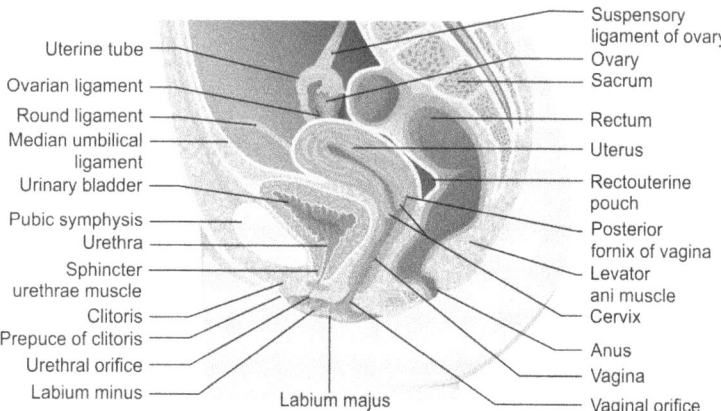

Figure 1.1: Female urogenital system (mid sagittal view through the pelvic cavity).

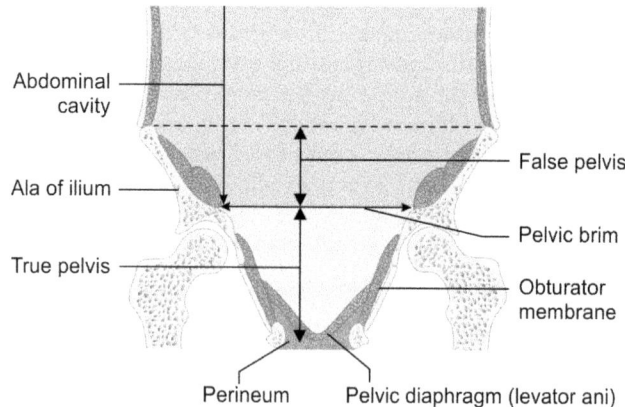

Figure 1.2: True and false pelvis.

Its boundaries are:
- Posteriorly—lumbar vertebrae
- Laterally—iliac fossa
- Anteriorly—anterior abdominal wall.

True Pelvis (Obstetric Pelvis)[3,4]

The true pelvis constitutes the bony canal which the fetus has to negotiate during delivery. The parts of true pelvis (Fig. 1.3) are:
- Pelvic inlet
- Pelvic cavity/mid plane
- Pelvic outlet.

Planes: The plane of the pelvic brim in the erect posture forms an angle of 60° with the horizontal. The axis of the birth canal is J-shaped and called the "Curve of Carus".[2]

Pelvic shape: Male and female pelvic cavity are different. Shape of female pelvic cavity is cylindrical. It is narrowest between the two ischial spines. There are four basic shapes of the pelvis recognized and described by Caldwell-Moloy (Table 1.1 and Fig. 1.4). Mixed forms also exist.[3-5]

BLOOD SUPPLY OF THE PELVIC ORGANS[4,6]

At the L4 level abdominal aorta divide into right and left common iliac artery. From the L4 level it will descend down to the pelvic area and again it will divide into external and internal iliac artery. At the pelvic area, internal iliac artery will branch into anterior and posterior part and supply blood to the pelvic organs, perineum region and muscles of gluteal area. Most of the blood supply of pelvic organs is from the anterior division

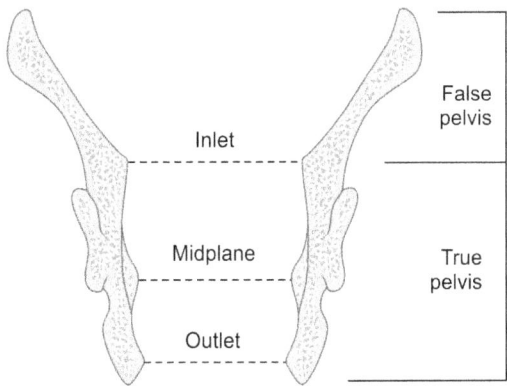

Figure 1.3: Parts of true pelvis.

Table 1.1: Classification of female pelvis by Caldwell-Moloy.

Parameter	Pelvic Shapes			
	Gynecoid	Android	Anthropoid	Platypelloid
Configuration	Normal	Male type	Ape type	Flat pelvis
Incidence	42%	32%	23.5%	2.5%
Brim shape	Rounded	Heart shape	Long oval	Flat oval
Mid pelvis				
Sacrum	Wide, curved	Narrow, flat	Long, narrow	Wide, curved
Side walls	Parallel	Funneled	Straight	Parallel
Ischial spines	Not prominent	Prominent	Variable	Variable
Sacrosciatic notch	Short and wide	Narrow and long	Wide	Short
Depth	Average	Long	Long	Short
Pelvic outlet				
Pubic arch	Wide	Narrow	Narrow	Very wide
Effect on labor				
Outcome	Average sized baby, good prognosis	Deep transverse arrest, obstetric assistance	Face to pubes delivery	Delay at inlet only

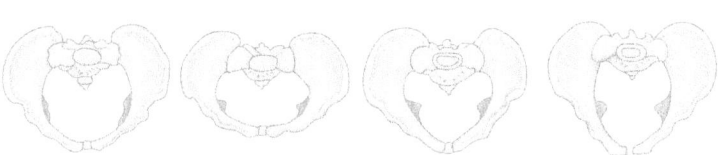

Gynecoid   Platypelloid   Android   Anthropoid

Figure 1.4: Classification of female pelvis by Caldwell-Moloy.

of internal iliac artery. Posterior division of internal iliac artery supplies blood to the gluteal region.

The external iliac arteries will divide into two branches named inferior epigastric artery and deep circumflex iliac artery to supply lower extremities (Fig. 1.5).

Branches of Anterior Division of Internal Iliac Arteries Supplies

- Upper part of bladder is supplied by the umbilical and superior vesical artery. Rectum is supplied by the middle rectal artery.
- Muscles of pelvic area are supplied by the obturator artery.
- Anal muscles, perineal muscles and skin are supplied by the internal pudendal artery.
- Uterus, fallopian tube, ovary and vagina are supplied by the uterine artery. The branch of this artery which supplies vagina is also known as vaginal artery.

The veins will accompany all these arteries and it will return the deoxygenated blood back.

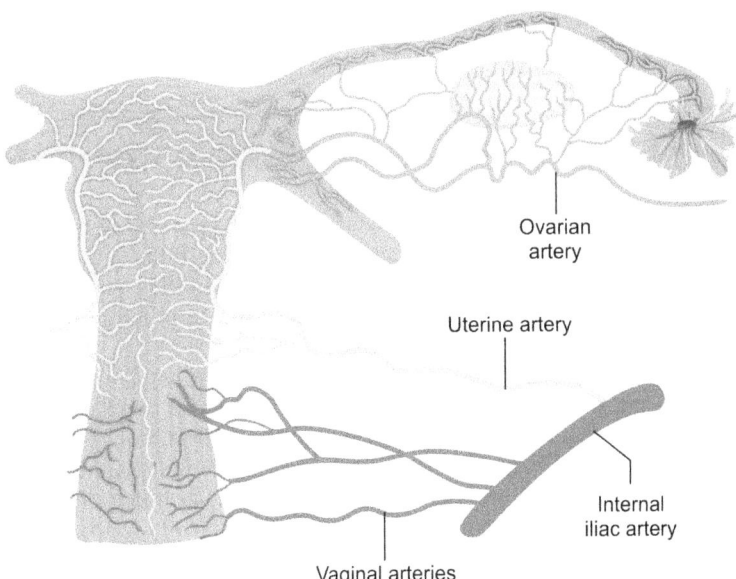

Figure 1.5: Blood supply of the pelvic organs.

LYMPHATIC DRAINAGE OF THE PELVIS[4]

External and internal iliac lymph nodes and sacral lymph nodes receive lymph from the pelvic organs. Internal iliac lymph nodes also receive lymph from the perineum and gluteal region. Common lymph nodes will receive lymph from the other lymph nodes.

Pelvic lymph nodes are connected to each other. It means that the cancer cells can easily spread to pelvic area and if nodes are removed as a part of treatment, the removal will not disturb the lymphatic drainage.

NERVE SUPPLY OF THE PELVIS

Pelvis is innervated by sacral and coccygeal plexus and pelvic part of autonomic nervous system.

Sacral and coccygeal plexus: Sacral plexus is formed by lumbosacral trunk (L4, L5), ventral rami of S1-S3 and the upper division of S4. It is present in the front of the piriformis and supply buttocks, lower limb and structures of pelvis. Largest branch of sacral plexus is sciatic nerve.

The coccygeal plexus is interconnected with the lower part of sacral plexus. It originates from the S4, S5, Co 1 spinal nerves. The only nerve in this plexus is anococcygeal nerve which supplies the skin over the coccyx.[4]

Pudendal Nerve and its Importance in Obstetric Practice[4,7]

The pudendal nerve is the chief nerve of perineum and external genitalia.

Origin: It originates from sacral plexus in the pelvis, S2, S3 and S4 nerve roots.

Course: It originates in the pelvis, enters into gluteal region through greater sciatic notch and leaves through lesser sciatic notch. Then it enters into posterior part of pudendal canal and gives off the inferior rectal nerve. Inferior rectal nerve will further divides into two terminal branches, perineal nerve and dorsal nerve of clitoris.

In obstetric practice, pudendal nerve block is administered while conducting vaginal delivery to render the vulva and perineal areas numb. Pudendal nerve block along with local infiltration of the labia majora achieves adequate anesthesia for spontaneous vaginal delivery with or without episiotomy, for conducting vaginal instrumental assisted delivery (low forceps, vacuum extraction), breech delivery and for repair of episiotomy and perineal tears or lacerations.

Pelvic part of autonomic nervous system: Sympathetic nervous system reach the plexus by downward continuation of sympathetic trunks and aortic plexus.

CHANGES IN MAMMARY GLANDS DURING PREGNANCY

Giving birth to a baby is not an easy thing. It makes many changes in woman's body. Hormonal change is one of it. Woman's body will change and prepare to feed her baby. For this feeding purpose, her breasts also known as mammary glands will change. In response to ovarian hormone, mammary glands develop in females. It is exocrine and modified sweat glands produce milk for the baby.

Mammary gland is made up of hollow cavities lined with epithelial and myoepithelial cells known as alveoli and has 15 – 20 lobes. Alveoli will join with each other and form lobules. Lobule has milk producing duct which opens in the nipple. The myoepithelial cells can contract and relax similar to muscle cells, and thereby push the milk towards the nipple, where it collects in sinuses of the ducts. A suckling baby essentially squeezes the milk out of these sinuses.[8,9]

At the time of birth we don't have alveoli. Before puberty, due to the estrogen hormone alveoli will develop but it does not secret milk. During pregnancy, estrogen and progesterone levels will increase. Increased level of these hormones will increase the adipose tissue and blood flow to the mammary glands and the secretary alveoli will develop. When baby sucks the nipple it causes the release of oxytocin hormone and stimulates the contraction of myoepithelial cells. This helps to release the milk.[3,8,9]

Lymphatics drain into the axillary transpectoral and internal mammary glands. During pregnancy under the influence of various hormones like chorionic gonadotropins, estrogens, progesterone, cortisol, insulin, human placental lactogen, prolactin and thyroxin the breasts enlarge in size, there is increase in vascularity, increased pigmentation, formation of secondary areola and appearance of Montgomery's tubercles. A clear secretion can be generally expressed out of the nipples. During pregnancy the hormones prepare the breasts for the function of lactation by inducing mammogenesis, lactogenesis, galactokinesis and galactopoiesis (Fig. 1.6).[2]

Human Milk[10]

Milk secreted at the end of pregnancy and immediately after delivery is rich in fat and immunoglobulines. It is known as colostrums. Otherwise

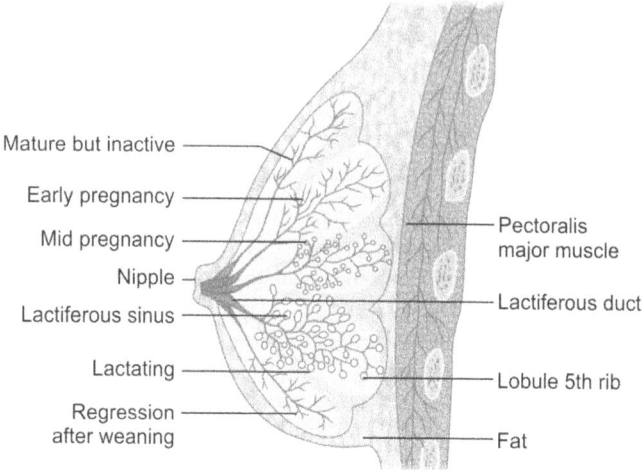

Figure 1.6: Changes in female breast during pregnancy.

the milk is composed of 88% of water, 4% fat, 1% protein, ions, vitamins, IgA and lactose.

Newborn baby's breast may secrete milk during first week after birth. It is known as "witch's milk". Woman will produce milk for about 5-6 months after delivery and then diminishes progressively, so that the infant is weaned by about 9 months of age.

HORMONAL CONTROL OF OVULATION

Ovulation is a process mainly controlled by the interaction of hormones released from the hypothalamus and anterior pituitary with the hormones produced from reproductive tissue and organs. The hypothalamus regulates the release of hormones from the pituitary gland.

In female FSH and LH stimulates the development of ova (egg cells). It is developed as follicles. These follicles inhibit the FSH stimulation. It also plays a role in induction of ovulation and stimulates the production of estrogen and progesterone by ovaries. These two are steroid hormones which prepare the body for pregnancy.

Effects of female reproductive hormones are given in Table 1.2

FEMALE REPRODUCTIVE CYCLE

Female reproductive cycle includes ovarian and uterine cycles. Menstrual cycle is also known as uterine cycle. In this the cyclic changes occur in the endometrium of uterus.

Maternal Anatomy and Physiology

Table 1.2: Effects of female reproductive hormones.[11,12]

Hormone	Source	Effects
FSH (Follicle stimulating hormone)	Anterior pituitary (Adenohypophysis)	• Stimulates the growth and development of the follicle • Stimulates secretion of estrogen • Enhances effect of LH in stimulating ovulation
LH (Luteinizing hormone)	Anterior pituitary (Adenohypophysis)	• Stimulates the final development of the follicle • Stimulates ovulation • Stimulates the development of the corpus luteum • Stimulates production of progesterone
Estrogen	Preovulatory (Graafian) follicle	• Stimulates repair of uterine lining • At high concentration inhibits FSH, however during 'pituitary hormone surge' it stimulates further FSH production • As concentration peaks stimulates release of LH
Progesterone	Postovulatory follicle (Corpus luteum)	• Maintains uterine lining • Inhibits release of FSH • Inhibits release of LH • Fall in concentration results in menstruation • Fall in concentration removes inhibition of FSH and a new cycle begins

Every month, endometrium of uterus gets prepared for the arrival of fertilized ovum. This fertilized ovum will develop in the uterus and form fetus. But if the ovum is not fertilized, the lining if uterus will shed off. This shedding off of lining of endometrium accompanied by bleeding is known as Menstruation. Menstruation starts at puberty and stops permanently at menopause. First menstruation is known as menarche.[13]

Phases of the Menstrual and Ovarian Cycles

The menstrual (uterine) cycle begins with the first day of bleeding, and ends just before the next menstrual period. Thus the cycle continues menstrual cycles normally range from about 25 to 36 days. All the women will not have exactly 28 days of cycle. Only 10-15% of women have cycles that are exactly 28 days.

Menstrual Cycle[13,14]

Days 1–5: Menstrual Phase

- This phase is from first day of the menses to last day of bleeding (usually lasts from 3-5 days, up to 7 days). Bleeding occurs when there is no fertilization.
- Reduced level of progesterone and estrogen causes constriction of endometrial blood vessels and cutting of the blood flow to the uterine lining. So the cells of the uterine lining start to die. Progressively it will shed off with the bleeding. Around two third of the endometrial lining will shed off during the cycle.

Days 6–14: Proliferative Phase

- This phase is from cessation of menses to ovulation.
- Endometrial lining thickens in preparation for implantation of a fertilized ovum. Its thickness doubles to about 4-6 mm.
- Uterine secreting glands increase in size and produce mucus.
- Uterine blood vessels begin to grow.
- Ovulation occurs in the ovaries at the end of this stage, usually around day 14, triggered by a surge in luteinizing hormone (LH) from the anterior pituitary gland.

Days 15–28: Secretary Phase

- This phase is from ovulation to the start of the next menses.
- Endometrial glands secrete mucus, which prepares the uterus to receive a fertilized ovum.
- The corpus luteum produces estrogen, while the cells of the ovaries produce progesterone.
- Endometrium continues to thicken.

Ovarian Cycle[13]

While the uterus is proceeding through the three phases above, the ovaries pass through the following phases:

1. *Follicular phase (about 14 days)*: Between 3-30 follicles, each containing 1 ovum begins to grow with usually 1 reaching maturity while the others break down.

Maternal Anatomy and Physiology

2. *Ovulatory phase (about 16–32 hours)*: The ovum is released from the follicle and enters the fallopian tube.
3. *Luteal phase (about 14 days)*: The ruptured follicle forms a structure called the corpus luteum. The corpus luteum produces progesterone, which helps prepare the endometrium for a fertilized egg.

Fertile Days of the Menstrual Cycle (Fig. 1.7)

A woman's fertile days depend on ovulation as well as the life span of the ovum and the sperm. The ovum and sperm are most likely to join, and pregnancy is most likely to occur, when unprotected sexual intercourse takes place during the 2 days before ovulation or on the day of ovulation. It is also possible a day or 2 after ovulation although this is less likely. Most women ovulate between 11 and 16 days after the first day of their last period. This is the time when women are most fertile and most likely to get pregnant.[13]

ANATOMICAL AND PHYSIOLOGICAL CHANGES DURING PREGNANCY

During pregnancy, women experience both physical and emotional changes. These changes are normal and to be expected.

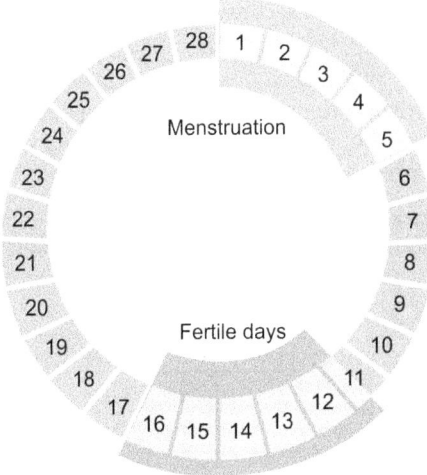

Figure 1.7: Fertile days of menstrual cycle.

Weight Gain during Pregnancy (Table 1.3)

In normal pregnancy, variable amount of weight gain is constant. In early weeks woman may lose weight due to nausea or vomiting. During subsequent months weight gain is progressive until the last 1 or 2 weeks. Total recommended weight gain during pregnancy is an average of 9 to 14 kg. This has been distributed to average 1 kg in first trimester and 5 kg in second and third trimester.[3,15]

Hematology

Blood Volume

There is an overall increase in plasma, red blood cell (RBC) and total blood volume. Plasma volume increases by 15% during the first trimester, accelerates in the second trimester, peaks at around 32 weeks reaching up to 50% above non-pregnant levels, and stays elevated until term. It returns to non-pregnant levels by 6 days post-delivery. There is often a sharp rise of up to 1 liter in plasma volume, within maternal circulation, 24 hours after delivery.[15, 16]

Increased requirements due to:
- Extra blood flow to uterus
- Metabolic needs of fetus
- Increased perfusion to other organs during pregnancy
- Blood loss in delivery:
  - Loss of 500–600 mL for vaginal delivery
  - Loss 1,000 mL for C-section.

Red Blood Cell Volume

Red blood cell (RBC) volume falls during the first 8 weeks of pregnancy, increasing back to non-pregnant levels by 16 weeks and then rising to 30% above non-pregnant levels by term. The relatively smaller increase

Table 1.3: Total weight gain for single fetus.[15,17]	
Fetus	3.36–3.88 kg
Placenta	0.48–0.72 kg
Amniotic fluid	0.72–0.97 kg
Uterus and breasts	2.42–2.66 kg
Blood and fluid	1.94–3.99 kg
Muscle and fat	0.48–2.91 kg Total: 9.70–14.55 kg

Maternal Anatomy and Physiology

in RBC compared with plasma results in hemodilution and "physiological anemia of pregnancy", which is not a true anemia but is representative of the greater increase of plasma volume. The increase in plasma volume occurs as a result of hormonal stimulation to meet the oxygen demands of pregnancy.[15,16]

Coagulation and Fibrinolysis in Pregnancy

Plasma levels of factors VII, VIII, IX, XII, together with fibrinogen and fibrin degradation products, increase during pregnancy (fibrinogen from 2.5 to 4 g/L). Factor XI and III decrease. These change increases coagulability and make pregnancy a 'hypercoagulable' state.

Platelets

Pregnancy is associated with increased platelet turnover. Thrombocytopenia (platelets <100 × 10^9/l) occurs in 0.8-0.9% of normal pregnant women, while increases in platelet factor and β thromboglobulin suggest elevated platelet activation and consumption. Since there is no change in platelet count in the majority of pregnant women, there is probably an increase in platelet production to compensate for the increased consumption.[16]

Principal blood changes during pregnancy are given in Table 1.4

Cardiovascular System

Heart

The heart size increases and is pushed upwards and rotated forwards, with lateral displacement of the left border.[15,16] All heart sounds are louder

Table 1.4: Principal blood changes during pregnancy.				
Parameters	Non-pregnant	Pregnancy near term	Total increment	Change
Blood volume (mL)	4,000	5,500	1,500	30–40% increase
Plasma volume (mL)	2,500	3,750	1,250	40–50% increase
Red cell volume (mL)	1,400	1,750	350	20–30% increase
Total Hb (g)	475	560	85	18–20% increase
Hematocrit (whole body)	38%	32%		Diminished

and the first sound is split. A systolic ejection murmur is normal and is due to turbulence secondary to increased blood flow through normal heart valves. A diastolic murmur is heard occasionally. Cardiac output is increased as a result of increased heart rate, reduced systemic vascular resistance and increased stroke volume.[16] Cardiac output increases 30% to 60% during pregnancy and is most significantly increased when a woman is in the left side-lying position, in which the uterus places the least pressure on the aorta.[15]

Heart rate is increased above non-pregnant values by 15% at the end of the first trimester.

This increases to 25% by the end of the second trimester, but there is no further change in the third trimester. Stroke volume is increased by about 20% at 8 weeks and up to 30% by the end of the second trimester, then remains level until term.[16]

Blood Pressure

Systolic blood pressure does not show a significant drop in pregnancy. It may drop slightly by 6–8%. However, there is a drop in diastolic pressure. It is reduced in the first two trimesters by up to 20–25% and returns to the non-pregnant level at term. This is due to the placenta acting as an arteriovenous shunt together with peripheral vasodilating factors such as estrogen, progesterone and increased endothelial synthesis of prostaglandin E2 and prostacyclins. Both blood pressure and cardiac output are reduced during epidural analgesia. In a supine position 70% of mothers have a fall in blood pressure of at least 10%, and 8% have decreases between 30 and 50%.[16]

Respiratory System

Anatomical Changes

Capillary engorgement of the nasal and pharyngeal mucosa and larynx begins early in the first trimester. This may explain why many pregnant women complain of difficulty in nasal breathing, experience more episodes of epistaxis and experience voice changes. The thoracic cage increases in circumference by 5–7 cm because of the increase in both the anteroposterior and transverse diameters from flaring of the ribs. The level of the diaphragm rises by about 4 cm early in pregnancy even before it is under pressure from the enlarging uterus. This would account for the decrease in residual volume since the lungs would be relatively compressed at forced expiration.[16]

Physiological Changes

During pregnancy minute ventilation increases by about 40% from 7.5 to 10.5 l/min and oxygen consumption increases by about 18% from 250 to 300 mL/min. Tidal volume increases gradually from the first trimester by up to 45% at term. Functional residual capacity is decreased by 20-30% at term due to reductions of 25% in expiratory reserve volume and 15% in residual volume.[16]

Blood gases: $PaCO_2$ decreases to 3.7-4.2 kPa by the end of the first trimester and remains at this level until term. Metabolic compensation for the respiratory alkalosis reduces the serum bicarbonate concentration to about 18-21 mmol/L, the base excess by 2-3 mmol/L and the total buffer base by about 5 mmol/L. PaO_2 in upright pregnant women is in the region of 14.0 kPa, higher than that in non-pregnant women. This is due to lower $PaCO_2$ levels, a reduced arteriovenous oxygen difference and a reduction in physiological shunt. Pregnant women maintain a normal arterial pH of 7.4 to 7.45.[16]

Renal System

Kidney size increases by about 1 cm in length. There is marked dilatation of renal calyces, pelvis and ureters. Increase in glomerular filtration rate (GFR) by about 50% reaches maximum at the end of first trimester and is maintained at this augmented level until at least the 36th gestational week. 24-hour creatinine clearance increases by 25% at 4 weeks after the last menstrual period and by 45% at 9 weeks. During the third trimester a consistent and significant decrease towards non-pregnant values occurs preceding delivery.[16]

Gastrointestinal System

Gums may swell and bleed easily. Incidence of dental caries is increased. Barrier pressure (lower esophageal sphincter (LOS) pressure minus gastric pressure) is reduced significantly during pregnancy compared with the non-pregnant state, due to increased intragastric pressure and reduced LOS pressure. LOS pressure appears to return to normal by 48 hours post-delivery.[16]

Endocrine System

Glucose Metabolism

Pregnancy is associated with an insulin-resistant condition, similar to that of type II diabetes. Early in pregnancy, increasing estrogen and progesterone levels, which lead to pancreatic cell hypertrophy and insulin excretion, alter maternal carbohydrate metabolism. Secretion of other hormones such as human placental lactogen, prolactin, cortisol, estrogen and progesterone induce insulin resistance. These hormones are found to be in significantly greater levels in pregnant women.[10]

Thyroid

There is increased synthesis of thyroxine binding globulin (TBG) by the liver in pregnancy. This increase leads to a compensatory rise in serum concentrations of total T4 and T3. There is, however, no change in the amount of free circulating thyroid hormones. There is iodine deficiency as a result of loss through increased glomerular filtration and decreased renal tubular absorption. Active transport of iodine to the fetoplacental unit and fetal thyroid activity also deplete the maternal iodide pool further from the second trimester.

Pituitary

There is significant enlargement of the pituitary gland during pregnancy. The growth is as a result of increase in the number of prolactin-secreting cells, with the proportion of lactotrophs increasing from 1% to 40%. This results in elevated prolactin levels to up to 10–20 times those of normal, non-pregnant values. These will return to normal by 2 weeks postpartum, unless the woman breastfeeds. Gonadotrophin levels are suppressed by the high concentrations of estrogen and progesterone and are undetectable during pregnancy. Levels of basal growth hormone and antidiuretic hormone remain unchanged during pregnancy.

Adrenal

Plasma CBG (corticosteroid binding globulin) concentrations increase during pregnancy. Levels of both free and bound cortisol also increase and levels of serum and urinary free cortisol increase three-fold by term. Adrenocorticotropic hormone (ACTH), which influences steroid secretion from adrenal cortex, remains within the normal range for non-pregnant women.

Skin

During pregnancy the skin undergoes a number of changes, mainly due to hormonal changes.

Pigmentation: Hyper pigmentation occurs in up to 90% of women during pregnancy. This begins in the first trimester and is prominently noticed in areas of normal hyperpigmentation such as nipples, areola, perineum and vulva. Both estrogens and progesterone, which have melanogenic stimulant properties, are responsible for this hyperpigmentation.

Linea nigra: This appears as an area of pigmentation extending from symphysis pubis to xiphisternum. Although the pigmentation fades after delivery it rarely returns to prepregnancy levels.

Melasma: Develops in up to 70% of women, mainly in the second half of pregnancy. It appears as patches of light-brown facial pigmentation usually over the forehead, cheeks, upper lip, nose and chin.

Spider naevi: These present as a central red spot and reddish extensions which radiate outwards like a spider's web and occur on the face, the trunk and arms. Most appear in early pregnancy and regress following delivery, although in up to 25% of women they may persist. Recurrences are known to occur at the same site in subsequent pregnancies.

Striae gravidarum: They appear perpendicular to skin tension lines as pink linear wrinkles. They fade and become white and atrophic, although never disappear completely.

Palmar erythema: Palmar erythema is reddening of the palms at the thenar and hypothenar eminences. This is due to high levels of estrogen in pregnancy and is seen in up to 70% of women by the third trimester and fade within 1 week of delivery.

Anatomical and physiological changes in pregnancy are given in Table 1.5.

PELVIC FLOOR MUSCLES

Pelvic floor is a funnel or dome-shaped muscular sheet which separates the pelvic cavity from the anatomical perineum.

The pelvic floor is composed of both muscles and connective tissue. The muscles are the active components that are through their contractions responsible for all functions of the pelvic floor. The connective tissues, with their elastic and collagen fibers and their extracellular matrices, provide structural support for the vagina and other organs such as uterus, urethra, bladder and rectum. Upper surface of pelvic floor is concave and slopes downwards, backwards and medially and it is covered by parietal layer of pelvic fascia. The inferior surface is convex and it is covered by anal fascia. The muscle with the covering fascia is known as "Pelvic Diaphragm".[3,18]

The pelvic floor consists of three muscle layers:[7]
- Superficial perineal layer (Nerve supply pudendal nerve)
    - Bulbocavernosus
    - Ischiocavernosus
    - Transversus perinei superficialis

Table 1.5: Anatomical and physiological changes in pregnancy.[16]

Parameters		<12 weeks	13–28 weeks	29 weeks
Hematological parameters	Plasma volume	↑10–15%	Further rise (gradual)	↑50%
	Red cell volume	Falls	Reaches 'non-pregnant' Levels	↑30%
	Total blood volume	↑10%	↑30%	↑45%
	Platelet count	→/↓	→/↓	↓0–5%
	Hemoglobin	↓	↓	↓15%
	White blood cell (WBC)/ erythrocyte sedimentation rate (ESR)	→/↑	→/↑	↑
	Factors V, VII, VIII, IX, XII, fibrinogen, vWF	→/↑	→/↑	↑
	Prothrombin III, protein C, protein S, plasminogen activator inhibitor	→/↓	→/↓	↓
Cardiovascular physiology	Heart rate	↑15%	↑30%	↑30%
	Stroke volume	↑20%	↑30%	↑30%
	Cardiac output	↑30–40%	↑30–50%	Remains over 50%
	Systolic and diastolic blood pressure	↓	→/↑	Non-pregnant value
Respiratory changes	Tidal volume	↑	↑	↑45
	Functional residual capacity (FRC)			↑20–30%
	Inspiratory reserve volume (IRV)			↑5%

Contd...

Maternal Anatomy and Physiology

Contd...

Parameters		<12 weeks	13–28 weeks	29 weeks
	Expiratory reserve volume (ERV)			↑25%
	Total lung capacity (TLC)			↓0–5%
Renal system	Glomerular filtration rate (GFR)	↑50%		Declines gradually
	Creatinine clearance	↑45%		Steady↓ towards non-pregnant values
	Glycosuria			↑
	Proteinuria			↑
Gastrointes-tinal	Lower esophageal sphincter (LOS) pressure	↓	↓	↓
	Gastric acid secretion			↓
	Gastric emptying			↓
	Heartburn			↓

- ❖ Deep urogenital diaphragm layer (Nerve supply pudendal nerve)
  - Compressor urethrae
  - Sphincter urethrae
  - Sphincter urethrovaginalis
- ❖ Pelvic diaphragm (Nerve supply sacral nerve roots S3 – S5)
  - Levator ani: Pubococcygeus (pubovaginalis, puborectalis), iliococcygeus
  - Coccygeus / Ischiococcygeus
  - Piriformis
  - Obturator internus.

Pelvic Floor during Pregnancy and Parturition

During pregnancy levator muscles becomes less rigid and more distensible. Studies also shown that levator muscle get hypertrophied during pregnancy. Due to water retention it swells and sags down. In second stage, the puborectalis and pubovaginalis muscles relax and levator ani is drawn up over the advancing presenting part in the second stage. Failure of levator ani to relax at the crucial moment may leads to extensive damage of pelvic structures.[3] It has been shown, that connective tissue changes occur during pregnancy. Weakening of collagen cross bonding added to dilatation of the vaginal canal at childbirth can lead to over-distension or rupture of connective tissue. The first vaginal birth is especially associated with the development of a prolapse, whereas additional vaginal births do not show significant increases in the odds of prolapsed.[18-21]

STUDY QUESTIONS

1. Explain about the obstetric pelvis and write in detail about classification of female pelvis by Caldwell-Moloy.
2. Which of the following is the least likely physiological change in pregnancy?
   a. Increase in intravascular volume
   b. Increase in cardiac output
   c. Increase in stroke volume
   d. **Increase in peripheral vascular resistance**
      (There is decrease in peripheral vascular resistance during pregnancy).

REFERENCES

1. Scanlon VC, Sanders T. Essentials of Anatomy and Physiology, 5th edition. FA Davis Company: United States of America; 2007.
2. Singh V. Textbook of Anatomy Abdomen and Lower Limb, 2nd edition, Vol 2. Reed Elsevier India Private Limited: New Delhi; 2014.
3. Dutta DC, Konar H. DC Dutta's Textbook of Obstetrics, 8th edition. Jaypee Brothers Medical Publishers: New Delhi; 2015.
4. Daftary SN, Chakravarti S. Manual of Obstetrics, 3rd edition. Reed Elsevier India Pvt. Ltd: New Delhi; 2011.
5. Kolesova O. Female pelvic types and age differences in their distribution. Institute of Anatomy and Anthropology, Papers on Anthropology XXI, 2012, pp. 147-54.
6. Fairley DH. Obstetrics and Gynecology, 2nd edition. Blackwell Publishing:London; 2004.
7. Seshayyan S. Inderbir Singh's Textbook of Anatomy, 6th edition, Vol 2. Jaypee publication; 2016.
8. Breast changes during and after pregnancy. Breast Cancer Care – The Breast Cancer Care Support Charity, 4th edition. London; 2014.

9. Human Physiology/The Female Reproductive System, Page Number: 1–25.
10. Chaurasia BD. Human Anatomy, 5th edition, Volume 1. CBS Publishers;2013.
11. Reproduction and its Hormonal Control. Biology Mad, JG January 2004, pp.1-5.
12. Pelvic floor ultrasound: A review, Hans Peter Dietz.
13. Preservice Education Family Planning Reference Guide, Reproductive System and the Menstrual Cycle. pp.37-50.
14. Knobil and Neill's Physiology of Reproduction, 3rd edition, Volume 2, Elsevier Publication.
15. Kisner C, Colby LA. Therapeutic Exercise–Foundations and Techniques, 5th edition. Margaret Biblis Publishers: Philadelphia; 2007.
16. Yanamandra N, Chandraharan E. Anatomical and Physiological Changes in Pregnancy and their Implications in Clinical Practice. Cambridge University Press, pp.1-8.
17. Diana Hemilton Fairley, Obstetrics and Gynecology, 2nd edition, Blackwell Publisher.
18. Lied B, Markovsky O, Gunnemann A. The Role of Altered Connective Tissue in the Causation of Pelvic Floor Symptoms, Germany. pp. 1-20.
19. Agarwal S. Anatomy of Pelvic Floor and Anal Sphincters. JIMSA. 2012;25(1);19-21.
20. Raizada V, Mittal RK. Pelvic Floor Anatomy and Applied Physiology. Elsevier Inc; 2008, pp. 493-509.
21. Sudha Seshayyan, Inderbir Singh's Textbook of Anatomy, Jaypee Publication, Volume two, 6th edition, 2016.

CHAPTER 2

Maternal Biomechanics

> **Chapter Outline**
> ➤ Center of Gravity
> ➤ Changes in Spine and Pelvis
> ➤ Posture
> ➤ Gait

INTRODUCTION

Pregnancy is unique time in life of women with many physiological, morphological and hormonal changes affecting the musculoskeletal system. These changes may affect the balance and stability and can cause pain and discomfort. One of the most significant changes is body weight gain which should be from 9 to 14 kg in for the fetus to develop properly. Increasing of the body weight with every month of pregnancy is mainly related to growing of the fetus, uterus, placenta and the amount of amniotic fluid. The greatest increase of the body mass in the second and third trimester of the pregnancy occurs in the trunk area. It can cause muscle weakness and shifting of body's center of gravity. Abdominal muscles will get stretched and weak due to increased body mass in abdominal area.

Under the influence of relaxin hormone, tendons and ligaments get relaxed and joint mobility also increases. These changes lead to postural and gait changes from the second trimester of pregnancy. Franklin et al. compared the body posture in the first and third trimester of pregnancy and the result was increase in lumbar lordosis and anteversion of pelvis.[1-5]

CENTER OF GRAVITY

Center of gravity (COG) usually shifts upwards and anteriorly because of enlargement of uterus and breasts. So it puts extra strain on muscles and ligaments supporting vertebral column. Shift of COG requires postural compensations to maintain balance. By postural compensations, woman will try to maintain COG more posterior.

CHANGES IN SPINE AND PELVIS

Pregnancy causes considerable compensatory changes in mechanics and structure of spine and pelvis and so prepare for the delivery. Because of shift in COG, body will make postural compensations to maintain balance and that will lead to changes in spinal alignment.[1,6]

- To compensate shift in COG, cervical and lumbar lordosis increases and as sequential changes of this, anterior pelvic tilt occurs.
- Overstretching of rhomboids and back muscles causes increase in Lumbar lordosis and thoracic kyphosis.
- Knees hyperextension to compensate for shift in COG.
- Round shoulder and upper back, scapular protraction and shoulder internal rotation because of breast enlargement.
- Weight shifts towards heels to bring COG posterior. This can lead to "Waddling gait".

The posterior weight-bearing during pregnancy can produce lumbar disc changes. There is high tensile stress on anterior disc, constant increase in compression stress and increases intradiscal pressure on posterior disc. These changes can also aggravate by water retention during pregnancy and so disc pressure increases. It can further cause disc protrusion and then cord or nerve irritation and pain.

Biomechanics of Lumbar Spine during Pregnancy

Vertebral bodies in lumbar spine are larger than cervical and thoracic spine, which allows them to accommodate added weight and stress when a person is in an upright posture. The functional units of the vertebral bodies can be divided into anterior and posterior portions. The anterior portion composed of the vertebral bodies and the intervertebral discs between them. It provides support and weight-bearing strength as well as shock absorption. The posterior portion of the functional unit, which is the non-weight-bearing portion, includes vertebral foramen and it protects the spinal cord. It also contains the facet joints, which are diarthrodial joints. Same as all other diarthrodial joints in the body, facet joints have a joint cavity between the articulating bones and they are freely moveable. Role of facet joints is to direct movements of the functional unit as a whole in flexion, extension, and lateral flexion. Because of the large amount of body mass and lordotic curve at lumbar spine, the load and shearing forces acting on the lumbar spine are greater than those on the cervical and thoracic spine. Because of these factors, there are more chances of degenerative changes and disc herniation at lumbar spine.

During pregnancy, a woman develops postural changes that are necessary to maintain balance in the upright position. The increasing weight is distributed mainly in the woman's abdominal girth. After 12 weeks of pregnancy, the uterus can no longer be contained within the pelvis and the abdominal mass moves superiorly and anteriorly. Due to this change, abdominal muscles get stretched and weak and so they lose their ability to maintain neutral posture (Fig. 2.1).

During pregnancy, relaxin hormone increases ten times and reaches its peak between weeks 38 and 42. Relaxin creates joint laxity which is important for accommodation of enlarging uterus during pregnancy and also during labor. Joint laxity is more in multiparous women than in nulliparous women. Maximum laxity is notable in the anterior and posterior longitudinal ligaments, which reduces the ability to give static support in the lumbar spine. Due to this, chances of pain coming from facet joints and disc related problems are more. In the pelvis, symphysis pubis and sacroiliac joints has maximum joint laxity which will increase more during pregnancy. Symphysis pubis will continue to widen to a maximum of approximately 12 mm (normal width 0.5 mm) which eventually can cause vertical displacement of pubis and puts rotator stress on the sacroiliac joints.

The sacroiliac joints are stable joints. They have anterior and posterior tight ligamentous structures as well as a curved and sigmoid articular surface that limits movement. Movement in the sacroiliac joint will

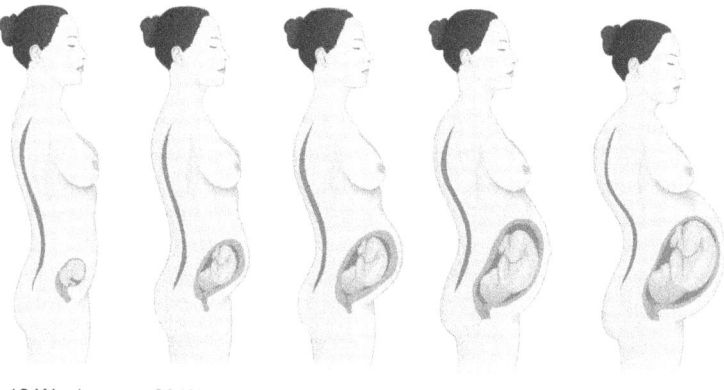

Figure 2.1: Postural changes during pregnancy. Note increasing lordosis of lumbar spine and increasing curvature of thoracic area. Abdominal mass moves superiorly and anteriorly.

increase throughout pregnancy. This movement can stretch pain-sensitive structures, and cause sacroiliac pain.

POSTURE

Normal pregnancy is accompanied by weight gain, increase in weight distribution in breasts and abdomen and softening of ligaments and connective tissue. Location of COG also changes because of increase of weight anteriorly. Consequently postural changes will occur to maintain balance and stability. Postural changes include:

- Chin and neck are pulled forward.
- Protraction of shoulder girdle
- Increase in cervical and lumbar lordosis
- Increased thoracic kyphosis
- Anterior pelvic tilt (The most common cause of lower back pain in most of the women)
- Knee hyperextension.

Franklin and Conner Kerr evaluate 12 pregnant women in first trimester and third trimester. They found changes in lumbar angle, head position and anterior pelvic tilt. Lumbar angle increased by an average of 6° and anterior pelvic tilt increased by an average of 4° head become more posterior as pregnancy progresses. These changes in posture will help to maintain center of mass which is centered over the base of support.[7]

GAIT

During pregnancy woman will walk with "Waddling gait", the wider base of support and increased external rotation of hip. Lumbar lordosis and proximal muscle weakness will contribute to waddling type of gait. This can become habitual and can continue after the delivery also (Table 2.1).

Woman will have slower gait with a decrease in walking frequency and stride length and increased step variability. These parameters are modified in order to promote safety during pregnancy. Double support time increases compared to single support time. These are fine adjustments that minimize the time on one leg to reduce muscle solicitation. Thus pregnant woman exaggerate transition phase to increase security of gait.[7]

During pregnancy, use of hip extensors, abductors and plantar flexors increases due to attempts to maintain normal stride length, cadence and joint angles. According to studies, the overuse of these muscle groups can contribute to development of low back and pelvic girdle pain, and other overuse injuries, commonly in women who have lower level of muscle strength and tight muscles before pregnancy. Women will try to maintain

Table 2.1: Gait parameters observed during pregnancy.	
Type of gait	Waddling gait
Base of support	Increased
Stride length	Decreased
Step width	Increased
Double support time	Increased
Single support time	Decreased
Velocity	Decreased
Cadence	Decreased

normal gait pattern but, stride length will decrease between second and third trimester because of greater lower trunk inertia. It will restrict trunk rotation in transverse plane. During third trimester, there will be increase in stance phase time, step width and double support time. Increased double support time will compensate for requirement of increased hip abductor muscle power during single limb support time in pregnancy. Increase in step width will cause lateral displacement of center of mass during walking which is referred as "waddling gait". Center of pressure at foot will move laterally. Contact time and gait velocity decreases. Gait cycle time is longer and the gait cycle was modified by an increase time of stance phase and a decrease of swing phase.[6-8]

STUDY QUESTIONS

1. Describe about the biomechanical changes in spine during pregnancy.
2. Describe about the pregnancy posture and relation of COG with posture and balance.
3. Posture correction in pregnancy.
4. Biomechanics of female pelvis.
5. Postural changes in pregnancy includes:
   a. Lumbar lordosis
   b. Protraction of shoulder girdle
   c. Hyperextension of knee
   d. **All of above**.

REFERENCES

1. Kisner C, Colby LA. Therapeutic Exercise – Foundations and Techniques, 5th edition. Margaret Biblis Publishers: Philadelphia; 2007.
2. Opala-Berdzik A, Bacik B, et al. Biomechanical Changes in Pregnant Women. 2009; 51- 5.

3. Branco M, Santos-Rocha R, Vieira F, et al. Biomechanics of gait during pregnancy. Sci World J. 2014;1-5.
4. Forczek W, Staszkiewicz R. Changes of kinematic gait parameters due to pregnancy, Volume 14(4). University School of Physical Education in Krakow: Poland; 2012, pp.113-9.
5. Madhuri GB. Textbook of Physiotherapy for Obstetrics and Gynecological Conditions. Jaypee Brothers Medical Publisher: New Delhi; 2007.
6. Bertuit J, Feipel V, Rooze M. Temporal and spatial parameters of gait during pregnancy. Acta Bioeng Biomech. 2015;17 (2):93-101.
7. Levangie PK, Norkin CC. Joint Structure and Function: A Comprehensive Analysis, Fourth edition. FA Davis Company, 2011.
8. Fitzgerald CM, Segal NA. Musculoskeletal health in pregnancy and postpartum: an evidence based guide for clinicians. Springer International Publishing; 2015.

CHAPTER 3

Approach to the Patient

Chapter Outline
- Diagnosis of Pregnancy
- Antenatal Assessment
- Postnatal Assessment

DIAGNOSIS OF PREGNANCY[1,2]

During the First Trimester (First 12 Weeks)

Subjective signs:
- Amenorrhea—cessation of menstruation at 4th week
- Morning sickness (nausea and vomiting) from 4th to 14th week
- Breast discomfort (increased size, tenderness, vascularization and swollen areolas)
- Pollakiuria due to bladder irritability
- Fatigue.

Objective signs:
- Jacquemier's or Chadwick's sign—Due to increased vascularity, bluish discoloration of vagina, cervix and labia occurs which is visible from approximately the fourth weeks of pregnancy.
- Goodell's sign—It is probable sign of pregnancy, consist of softening of cervix occurs as early as sixth week.

Uterine signs:
- Size and shape
- Hegar's sign—Softening of lower uterine segment, present at second and third month of pregnancy, palpated during bimanual examination.
- Palmer's sign—regular rhythmic uterine contractions palpated during bimanual examination by 4–8 weeks.

Immunological tests:
- Home pregnancy tests depends on the detection of the antigen (hCG) present in the maternal urine available commercially. It is most commonly used week after the missed menstrual period
- Blood tests for hCG-used only in special cases like, ectopic pregnancy.

During the Second Trimester (13–28 Weeks)
- Woman begins to feel fetal movements (quickening/feeling of life) and in some cases, uterine contractions.
- *Ballottement*: It is the diagnostic technique using palpation. When we tape or push a floating fetus, first it moves away and then returns to touch the examiner's hand.
- Fetal heart rate can be heard
- Lower abdomen will enlarge progressively.
- Chloasma—pigmentation over forehead and cheek
- Breast changes (enlargement with prominent veins, Montgomery's tubercles are prominent and extended).
- Colostrum
- Vaginal examination—bluish discoloration and internal ballottement

Investigation:
- Sonography
- Magnetic resonance imaging (MRI)
- Home pregnancy tests
- Blood tests for hCG—used only in special cases like, ectopic pregnancy.

Signs of pregnancy are described in Table 3.1.

ANTENATAL ASSESSMENT

Patient Profile[1]
- Full name: It is useful for the identification purpose.
- Age (in years): The woman having her first pregnancy at or after the age of 30 is called "elderly primigravida". Extremes of age (teenage and elderly) are obstetric risk factors.
- Husband's name: It is useful for the identification purpose.
- Husband's age (in years): When paternal age is above 40 at the time of conception, there are chances of increased risk to fetal health like,
  - Stillbirth
  - Increased risk of birth defects in the development of skull, heart and limbs

Table 3.1: Signs of pregnancy.

Gestational age	Sign	Other possible causes
Presumptive signs		
3–4 weeks	Breast changes	Premenstrual changes, oral contraceptives
4 weeks	Amenorrhea	Stress, vigorous exercise, early menopause, endocrine problems, malnutrition
4–14 weeks	Nausea, vomiting	Gastrointestinal virus, food poisoning
6–12 weeks	Urinary frequency	Infection, pelvic tumors
12 weeks	Fatigue	Stress, illness
16–20 weeks	Quickening	Gas, peristalsis
Probable signs		
5 weeks	Goodell sign	Pelvic congestion
6–8 weeks	Chadwick sign	Pelvic congestion
6–12 weeks	Hegar sign	Pelvic congestion
4–12 weeks	Positive result of pregnancy test (serum)	Molar pregnancy choriocarcinoma
6–12 weeks	Positive result of pregnancy test (urine)	False-positive results may be caused by pelvic infection, tumors
16 weeks	Braxton Hicks contraction	Myomas, other tumors
16–28 weeks	Ballottement	Tumors, cervical polyps
Positive signs		
5–6 weeks	Visualization of fetus by ultrasound examination	No other causes
6 weeks	Fetal heart tones detected by ultrasound examination	
16 weeks	Visualization of fetus by radiographic study	
8–17 weeks	Fetal heart sounds detected by Doppler ultrasound	
17–19 weeks	Fetal heart sounds detected by fetal stethoscope	
19–22 weeks	Fetal movements palpated	
Late pregnancy	Fetal movements visible	

Approach to the Patient

- Autism spectrum disorders
- Schizophrenia
- Childhood acute lymphoblastic leukemia – a carcinogenic condition, results in abnormal white cell production.
- Marital status: Married/Unmarried/Divorced/Separated: It has an effect on woman's psychological status.
- Educational status: It is important for parental education about pregnancy, labor, child care and maternal care before and after pregnancy etc.
- Occupation: To rule out the high risk occupation and guide the parents accordingly.
- Type of family: It helps to plan the antenatal care and labor.
- Income: It helps to plan the antenatal care and labor.
- Obstetric score:
  - Gravida: It is defined as total number of conformed pregnancies woman had regardless of outcome.
  - Para: It is defined as total number of births woman had after 20 weeks of gestation.
    Studies shows nulliparous woman have higher blood pressure levels throughout pregnancy, higher risk of gestational hypertensive disorders and vascular complications. The intensity of pain also differs in nulliparous and multiparous woman. Nulliparous woman experience more severe pain during early and active labor and comparatively less in second stage of labor.
  - Abortion: Studies shows that woman who had abortion after 16 weeks in previous had premature deliveries in current pregnancy. So this history is important to take precautions and prevent premature delivery.
  - Medical termination of pregnancy (MTP)
  - Living.

Obstetric History

Present Obstetric History[1]

- Conformation of pregnancy: Yes/No
- When, where and how it was confirmed?
- What test was done for confirmation?
- Quickening: Generally it is felt around 17 weeks of pregnancy but it can take place anytime between 13 – 25 weeks of pregnancy. It helps to ensure baby's well being.
- Immunization: Give TT 2 or booster dose before 36 weeks of pregnancy and if not given then has to be given even after 36 weeks.

If pregnant woman has not received TT dose previously, give TT in labor (Table 3.2).
- Any other problems like vomiting, hemorrhoids, heart burn, backache, bleeding, varicose vein, constipation, leg cramps, fever, leucorrhea, anorexia, insomnia, other complaints.

Table 3.2: National Immunization schedule for pregnant woman.			
Vaccine	When to give	Route	Site
Tetanus toxoid–1	Early in pregnancy	Intramuscular	Upper arm
Tetanus toxoid–2	4 weeks after TT 1	Intramuscular	Upper arm
Tetanus toxoid–Booster	If received 2 TT doses in a pregnancy within last 3 years	Intramuscular	Upper arm

Past Obstetric History (Table 3.3)

Table 3.3: Record sheet of past obstetric history.								
Date of delivery	Place of delivery	Duration of pregnancy	Method of delivery	Course of pregnancy	Labor	Puer-perium	Baby	
							Gender	Weight

Menstrual History[1,3]

- Last normal menstrual period (LNMP): From the LNMP, expected date of delivery (EDD) has to be calculated
- Age of menarche
- Cycle duration
- Regularity
- Flow:
    - Heavy/moderate scanty
    - Clots
    - Number of days
- Any Dysmenorrhoea
- Relief measures: This relief measures can be used during labor for relaxation.
- Abnormal menstrual bleeding: Intermenstrual, post-coital.

Family History

Family history is important to rule out and prevent some genetic diseases and complications.
- Congenital diseases
- Any hereditary diseases
- Multiple pregnancy
- Diabetes
- Heart disease
- Any mental retardation.

Medical–Surgical History

- Childhood disease
- Chronic disease like asthma, diabetes, epilepsy
  - Asthma can get worst in pregnancy and it can also affect the fetus.
  - In case of diabetes, there are more chances of gestational diabetes which can lead to birth defects, stillbirth etc.
  - Pregnant woman who has epilepsy, deliver baby without any complications but if seizure occur during pregnancy, it can lead to fetal heart rate declaration, miscarriage due to trauma during seizure etc. Seizure not commonly occurs during labor.
- Previous surgery
- Injuries especially of back and pelvis
- Hepatitis
  - Acute viral hepatitis is the most common cause of jaundice in pregnancy.
  - Hepatitis A infection during second or third stage of labor can lead to preterm labor.
  - Maternal infection with hepatitis B or C, affects child at the time of birth. It can transmit to the baby in vaginal or cesarean section and can be prevented by proper medications during antenatal period and also during labor.
  - Hepatitis E infection in third trimester of pregnancy is most dangerous and it can lead to maternal and fetal morbidity and mortality.
- History of anemia
  - Helps to prescribe the medications and prevent the anemia during pregnancy. Anemia during pregnancy can lead to serious complications like low birth weight, premature birth and maternal mortality. Pregnant woman is at higher risk of developing anemia and in woman with history of anemia the risk is 5 times higher.

- Any medication taken at present or past
- Blood transfusion
- Allergic reaction.
  - During pregnancy, allergic reactions get worst so it is necessary to take precautions and avoid the allergens if possible. Pregnancy can also worsen the seasonal allergies like rhinitis. The cause of rhinitis is excess of hormones not the exposure to allergens.
- STD, HIV: If woman has STD or HIV during pregnancy, it can be transmitted to the fetus and can increase the chances of stillbirth, miscarriage or preterm delivery.

Nutrition

- General nutrition: Vegetarian/Nonvegetarian
- Appetite: Decreased/increased
- Any eating disorders.

Partner's Health History

- Blood type
- Genetic abnormalities: To rule out and prevent genetic complications and disorders.
- Chronic diseases
- Infections
- Use of drugs such as cocaine, alcohol: Use of drugs and alcohol during pregnancy increases the risk of birth defect, low birth weight babies, premature delivery and stillbirth. Studies shows that, consumption of cocaine, alcohol or tobacco during pregnancy results in brain structure changes in fetus which can persist into early adolescent.
- Smoking habits: Tobacco, cigarette. The chance of ectopic pregnancy is 20% higher in woman who smokes during pregnancy.
- Sexually transmitted disease: AIDS/HIV.

Gynecological Procedures

- Gynecological or abdominal surgery
- Previous ectopic pregnancies.

Physical Examination[4]

- General appearance
- Nourishment: Maternal nourishment is important to supply adequate nutrient to the fetus. If fetus will not get adequate nutrient it can lead to fetal malnutrition.

Approach to the Patient

- Body built: Ectomorphic/Mesomorphic/Endomorphic
- Height: Studies show that woman with shorter height (less than 160 cm) has more chances of caesarean section.
- Weight: Maternal obesity can increase the risk of preeclampsia, gestational diabetes, stillbirth and congenital anomalies.
- Vital signs:
  - Temperature
  - Pulse
  - Respiration
  - Blood pressure
- Mental status: Recent studies show that maternal anxiety in early pregnancy can increase the risk of ADHD in baby.
- Extremities:
  - Ankle edema: During pregnancy, extra fluid in the body and the pressure from the growing uterus can cause edema in the ankle and feet.
  - Capillary refill time: Apply pressure to an external capillary bed and then note the time taken for color to return. It is known as capillary refill time. Normal capillary refill time is less than 2 seconds. It is used to measure dehydration and the amount of blood flow to the tissue. Increased capillary refill time may indicate hypoxia, dehydration and anemia but further evaluation is needed to conform diagnosis.
  - Cyanosis
- Breast examination:
  - Any tenderness/painful
  - Tense/dilated veins/warmth/presence of crust
  - Nipples retracted/inverted/cracked
- Abdominal examination
- In the initial obstetric examination, speculum and bimanual pelvic examination is done:
  - To check for lesions or discharge
  - To note the color and consistency of the cervix
  - To obtain cervical samples for testing
- Pelvic examination:
  - Inspection of external genitalia
  - Rectovaginal examination
  - Rectal examination
  - Pelvic capacity can be tested by bimanual examination with the middle finger. Pelvic inlet is considered as adequate if the distance from the underside of the pubic symphysis to sacral promontory is more than 11.5 cm.

❖ Fetal heart rate and in patients presenting later in pregnancy lie of the fetus are assessed (Leopold maneuver).

Leopold Maneuver[3]

Palpation should be conducted with most gentleness. Purposeless palpation is uninformative and can cause undue uterine irritability. During Bratox-Hicks contraction or uterine contraction in labor, palpation should be suspended. The uterine fundus is palpated to determine which fetal part occupies the fundus. Each side of the maternal abdomen is palpated to determine which side is fetal spine and which the extremities are.

❖ **Fundal grip (Fig. 3.1A):**
  - Palpation is done facing the patient's face
  - Fundal area is palpated using both hands flat on maternal abdomen to find out which pole of the fetus is lying in the fundus
    - Broad, soft and irregular mass suggestive of breech
    - Smooth, hard and globular mass suggestive of head
    - In transverse lie neither of the fetal poles is palpated in the fundal area.

❖ **Lateral or umbilical grip (Fig. 3.1B):**
  - Palpation is done facing the patient's face
  - The hands are to be placed flat on either side of the umbilicus to palpate one after other, the sides and front of the uterus to find out the position of the back, limbs and the anterior shoulder
  - The back is suggested by smooth curved and resistant feel
  - The limb side is comparatively empty and there are small knobs like irregular parts
  - The position of the anterior shoulder forms a well marked prominence above the head.

❖ **Pawlik's grip (Fig. 3.1C):**
  - Palpation is done facing the patient's face
  - The overstretched thumb and four fingers of the right hand are placed over the lower pole of the uterus
  - Keep ulnar border of palm on the upper border of the symphysis pubis
  - When the fingers and the thumb are approximated, the presenting part is grasped distinctly. Side to side mobility is tested
  - In transverse lie powlik's grip is empty.

❖ **Pelvic grip (Fig. 3.1D):**
  - The examination is done facing the patient's feet
  - Four fingers of both the hands are placed on either side of the midline in the lower pole of uterus and parallel to the inguinal ligament

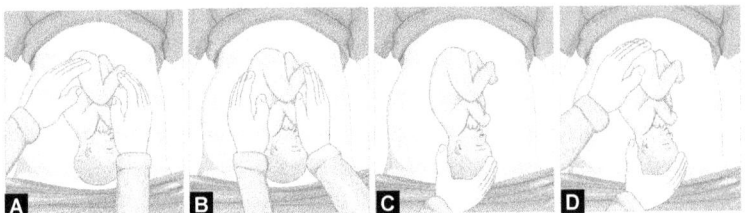

Figures 3.1A to D: Leopold maneuver: (A) Fundal grip; (B) Lateral grip; (C) Pawlik's grip; (D) Pelvic grip.

- The fingers are pressed downward and backward in a manner of approximation of finger tips to palpate the part occupying the lower pole of the uterus. Mobility from side to side is also tested
- Pelvic grip using both hands is favored as it is most comfortable for woman and also gives most information.

During subsequent visits, BP and weight assessment is important. Obstetric examination focuses on uterine size, fundal height (in cm above the symphysis pubis), fetal heart rate and activity, and maternal diet, weight gain, and overall well-being. Speculum or bimanual examination is usually not needed unless vaginal discharge or bleeding, leakage of fluid or pain is present.

Investigations

If a woman has Rh-negative blood, she may be at risk of developing Rh0 (D) antibodies, and the fetus may be at risk of developing erythroblastosis fetalis. Rh0 (D) antibody levels should be measured in pregnant women at 18–20 weeks and again at about 26–28 weeks.

Screening of gestational diabetes must be done between 24 and 28 weeks. If she is having any of the below risk factors, she must be screened during first trimester.

- Presence of gestational diabetes or macrosomic neonate. (Weight > 4.5 kg at birth in a previous pregnancy)
- Unexplained fetal losses
- A strong family history of diabetes in 1st-degree relatives
- A history of persistent glucosuria
- Body mass index (BMI) >30 kg/m^2
- Polycystic ovary syndrome with insulin resistance.

Calculation of the EDD[5,3]

The duration of pregnancy is usually 40 weeks, Normal labor occurs between 38 and 42 weeks. The formula for calculating expected date of delivery is known as Naegele's formula. Nine months plus seven days are added to the first date of the last menstrual period. Ovulation occurs 14 days after the first day of the last menstrual period.

Example:
The patient had her LNMP on 3rd January. Add 9 calendar months and 7 days to it. So 10th October becomes the EDD.

In case of IVF pregnancy, LMP date is 14 days prior to the date of embryo transfers.

POSTNATAL ASSESSMENT

Identification Data

- Name:
- Age:
- Hospital no:
- Marital status:
- Address:
- Husband's name:
- Occupation:
- Income:
- Date and time of admission:
- Date and time of delivery:

Present Obstetric History

- Parity: Nulliparous woman will have more perineal pain and sexual problems.
- Mode of delivery:
    - Normal vaginal
        - With episiotomy
        - Without episiotomy
        - Perineal tear: Perineal tears are classified into 4 categories: which are discussed in Table 3.4.
    - Spontaneous/Medical/Cesarean/Any other Woman who had cesarean delivery are commonly suffer from exhaustion and bowel problems. They have less perineal pain and lesser chances of urinary incontinence as compared to vaginal delivery.
    - Woman who had forceps or ventouse delivery will have more perineal pain as compared to unassisted vaginal delivery.
- Full term/premature.

Table 3.4: Perineal tear classification.	
1st degree tear	Laceration is limited to superficial perineal skin or vaginal mucosa
2nd degree tear	Laceration till perineal muscles and fascia
3rd degree tear	Perineal skin, vaginal mucosa, muscles, fascia and anal sphincter are torn
4th degree tear	Perineal skin, vaginal mucosa, muscles, fascia, anal sphincter and rectal mucosa are torn

Family History

Illness: Tuberculosis/hypertension/diabetes/asthma.

General Physical Examination[3]

- **Body built**:
- **Activity**:
- **Weight**:
- **Vital signs**:
  - Temperature:
  - Pulse:
  - Respiration:
  - Blood pressure:
- **Presence of**:
  - Palmar erythema:
  - Superficial varicosities:
  - Leg edema: Sites for evidence of edema are over the medial malleolus and anterior surface of the lower one-third of the tibia. The area is to be pressed with the thumb for at least 5 seconds.
  - Ankle edema: Slight degree ankle edema usually confined to one leg, more on the right.
    Dependent edema is physiological in pregnancy but generalized edema or facial edema can be first sign of disease.
  - Varicose veins:
- **Muscle testing:**
  - Muscles that tighten during pregnancy:
    - Hip flexors or Iliopsoas
    - Rectus femoris
    - Deep muscles of lower back (quadratus lumborum)
    - Pectorals
    - Internal rotators and elevators of shoulder, rhomboids, levator scapulae and the upper fibers of trapezius.

- Muscles that weaken or over stretch during Pregnancy:
  - Hip extensors or gluteals
  - Hamstrings
  - Abdominal muscles
  - Mid and lower fibers of trapezius in upper back
  - Shoulder external rotators
  - Serratus anterior.
- Neck flexors
- Pelvic floor muscles
- Intercostals.

Pelvic Floor Muscle Testing[6]

There are many grading scales to measure the strength of muscle but "Modified oxford scale" is the most commonly used scale. It is a six point scale. In this scale + and - can be added when a contraction is considered to fall between two full grades. So when the + and - both are used, the scale will expand to 15 point scale (Table 3.5).

❖ Diastasis recti muscle assessment (For detail check chapter 6: Postnatal Physiotherapy)
❖ Pelvic floor muscle assessment.
❖ Pelvic alignment: Assessment of pelvic girdle will identify biomechanical changes in alignment of pelvis and dysfunction. It can be the source of pain and discomfort during postnatal period.
❖ Postural assessment.

Table 3.5: Modified Oxford grading for pelvic floor muscle strength measurement.	
0	No contraction detected
1	Flicker
2	Weak: The patient is able to contract the pelvic floor muscles well enough to partially encircle the therapist's finger
3	Moderate: The patient is able to fully encircle the therapist's finger
4	Good: The patient is able to fully encircle the therapist's finger and partially pull the fingers further into the vaginal cavity
5	Strong: The patient is able to fully encircle the therapist's finger with a strong contraction and pull the finger fully up and into the vaginal canal

STUDY QUESTIONS

1. Write a short note about diagnosis of pregnancy.
2. Describe in detail about Leopold maneuver and its importance.
3. Naegele's formula and its importance.
4. Write a note on grading of pelvic floor muscles.
5. Antenatal screening tests.
6. Common symptoms of early pregnancy include all of the following, *except*:
   a. Nausea and vomiting
   b. Increased frequency of micturition
   c. Breast heaviness
   d. Abdominal enlargement
6. Which of the following should a woman avoid while she is pregnant?
   a. Smoking cigarettes
   b. Being under 20 and over 40 years of age
   c. Not having adequate prenatal medical supervision
   d. All of these

REFERENCES

1. Sved M. Gynecology. MCCQE 2002.
2. Coutin AS. Essential Obstetrics and Newborn Care. 2015.
3. Dutta DC, Konar H. DC Dutta's Textbook of Obstetrics. Jaypee Brothers Medical Publishers, 8th edition. 2015.
4. Hypertensive Disorders of pregnancy, Queensland Clinical Guidelines, Queensland Government, August 2015.
5. Essential Antenatal, Perinatal and Postpartum Care, WHO, Regional Office for Europe, February 2003.
6. Hislop HJ, Avers D, Brown M. Daniels and Worthingham's Muscle Testing: Technique of Manual Examination and Performance Testing, 9th edition, 2015.

CHAPTER 4

Antenatal Physiotherapy

> **Chapter Outline**
> ➢ Guidelines for Exercise during Pregnancy in Healthy Women
> ➢ Contraindications to Exercise during Pregnancy
> ➢ Benefits of Exercise during Pregnancy
> ➢ Routine Antenatal Care
> ➢ Exercises Prescription
> ➢ Antenatal Physiotherapy for First Trimester of Pregnancy
> ➢ Antenatal Physiotherapy for Second Trimester of Pregnancy
> ➢ Antenatal Physiotherapy for Third Trimester of Pregnancy
> ➢ Guidelines for Managing the Pregnant Women
> ➢ Sacroiliac Joint Pain/Posterior Pelvis Pain/Pelvic Girdle Pain
> ➢ Effects of Supine Lying during Pregnancy

INTRODUCTION

Pregnancy is physiological process and female body and organs can adjust to this process to maintain good maternal and fetal health. Antenatal care is an essential pillar of safe motherhood. Normal delivery is the best thing for mother and fetus as physiological point of view. There are many factors which lead to normal delivery and proper exercise is one of it. Beginning or continuing a moderate intensity exercise is beneficial for pregnant women and fetus.[1,12]

The aim is to give optimal care to the mother so that she can endure the nine months of pregnancy without any complications. Manual techniques, postural education, care of back and SI joint and ADL modification will help to reduce the joint stress in pregnant women. Physiotherapist should help the woman to activate transverse abdominus, multifidus and pelvic floor muscles which eventually helps to maintain the core stability, prevent back pain and SI joint pain and strengthen the core muscles.[2]

Postural adaptations such as forward shift, anterior pelvic tilt, increase in lumbar lordosis and thoracic kyphosis are common during pregnancy. 75% women shows more posterior posture, weight of the uterus is shifted posterior to the normal center of gravity which is the most common cause for back and pelvic pain during pregnancy.

Research shows that due to secretion of relaxin hormone, pre-pregnancy postural habits exaggerate during pregnancy which can cause back and pelvic pain. After the delivery of baby, woman will return to pre-pregnancy state. Therapist should educate pregnant women about the dangers of contact sports, scuba diving, fall and excessive joint stress which can result in fetal defects or fetal decompression disease.[1]

Travel

There is no specific contraindication to travel during pregnancy. The safest time to travel during pregnancy is between 14 and 28 weeks and she should always wear seat belt. Due to the risk of delivery in unfamiliar atmosphere, it is not safe to travel on airplanes after 34 weeks of gestation.

During any kind of travel, pregnant women should stretch and straighten their legs and ankles periodically to prevent venous stasis and the possibility of thrombosis.

Environment

Environmental condition is important during pregnancy as it affects the temperature regulation and hydration. For the hydration regulation, advice woman to take adequate fluids during and after exercise, avoid heat and humidity and wear loose fitting cloths.[3,6]

GUIDELINES FOR EXERCISE DURING PREGNANCY IN HEALTHY WOMEN[4,9,11,12,14,24]

- ❖ Obtain medical clearance before participation.
- ❖ The exercise prescription must be on the basis of individual needs and regular mild to moderate exercise is preferable with gradual increase in intensity.
- ❖ A maximum heart rate limit up to 155 b/min is recommended. It can be higher than this but only prescribed on an individual basis.
- ❖ Some recommended activities are walking, cycling, swimming, low impact aerobics and stretching.
- ❖ Exercise in supine position is not recommended after the 4th month due to possible risk of compression syndrome.

- Advice her not to stand steady for longer duration or perform exercises which can cause loss of balance.
- Drink plenty of fluids before, during and after exercise.
- Guide her to understand the warning signs to stop exercising and take rest when feels fatigued and never reach a point of exhaustion.
- Eat an additional 150-350 calories a day especially complex carbohydrates to replace muscle glycogen stores and to fulfill the additional nutritional demands.
- Must wear loose clothing which allows ventilation.
- Do not exercise in hot and humid climate or when feeling fatigued.
- Bouncy and jerky movements, high altitude activities and scuba diving should be avoided during pregnancy.
- Competitive contact sports are allowed only during the first 16 weeks of healthy pregnancy and only if woman was active in sports before pregnancy otherwise it must be avoided throughout pregnancy.
- Light to moderate weight lifting is encouraged to improve or maintain strength but Valsalva maneuver must be avoided.

CONTRAINDICATIONS TO EXERCISE DURING PREGNANCY (TABLE 4.1)

Table 4.1: Absolute and relative contraindications to exercise during pregnancy[5,6,9,11,14,19,24,26,29]

Absolute contraindications	Relative contraindications
Maternal cardiovascular, thyroid respiratory or systemic disease	History of 3 or more miscarriage or premature labor
Poor fetal growth	Maternal type I diabetes
Ruptured membranes–Rupture of amniotic fluid before the onset of labor or premature labor	History of rapid labor or poor fetal growth
Persistent bleeding after first trimester	Early pregnancy bleeding
Incompetent cervix, early dilatation of cervix before the pregnancy is full term.	Extremely sedentary lifestyle with very poor fitness
Preeclampsia: Pregnancy induced hypertension or toxemia	Breech presentation after 28 weeks
Multiple pregnancies (triplets, etc.)	Palpitations or arrhythmias
Placenta previa—placenta is located on the uterus in a position where it may detach before the baby is delivered	Anemia or iron deficiency

Contd...

Contd...

Absolute contraindications	Relative contraindications
Hemodynamically significant heart disease	Extreme over- or underweight
Restrictive lung disease	Chronic bronchitis
Sudden swelling of ankles hands and face	Extreme morbid obesity
Acute infectious disease	Extreme underweight
Risk for preterm labour	Orthopedic limitations
	Poorly controlled seizure disorder
	Heavy smoker

BENEFITS OF EXERCISE DURING PREGNANCY[14]

- It helps to avoid excessive fat accumulation and so maintains healthy body weight.
- Maintain or improve cardiovascular fitness, muscular strength and endurance, and flexibility.
- Helps to decrease or avoid the chances of musculoskeletal problems like back pain, SI pain and other minor discomforts of pregnancy.
- Improve posture and body mechanics, which will improve coordination, balance, and body awareness.
- Causes breathe awareness; enhance self image, reduce stress and gives relaxation.
- Prevent and treat gestational diabetes, hypertension, and preeclampsia.
- Helps to reduce the complications of delivery and promotes good and early postnatal recovery.

ROUTINE ANTENATAL CARE

Aims[8,15]

- To maintain and improve good physical and psychological health throughout the pregnancy.
- To identify and treat pregnancy complications.
- To detect fetal abnormalities as early as possible.
- To educate about pregnancy, labor, puerperium and care of newborn.

Subsequent Visits[15,29]

Following the first attendance it is most usual for women to be seen at interval of 4 weeks up to 28 weeks gestation, at interval of 2 weeks up to 36 weeks, and after that weekly till delivery. Always check for blood pressure, weight, presence of edema, fundal height and lie of the baby, fetal heart rate and movement.

Warning signs are:
- Leakage of fluid from vagina
- Vaginal bleeding
- Abdominal pain: Distressing in nature
- Headache
- Visual changes
- Decrease or loss of fetal movements
- Fever, rigor, excess vomiting and diarrhea.

Blood Pressure

Blood pressure must be checked at each antenatal visit. In early pregnancy, it is necessary to check baseline blood pressure. Initial recording of blood pressure before 12 weeks helps to differentiate a pre-existing chronic hypertension from a pregnancy induced hypertension developing later on. It slightly decreases during the second trimester due to dilatation of blood vessels. Increase in blood pressure can be the first sign of eclampsia.[10,15,28,29]

Maternal Weight Gain

In normal pregnancy, variable amount of weight gain is constant phenomenon. Initially woman may lose weight because of nausea and vomiting. During subsequent months weight gain is progressive until the last 1 or 2 weeks. This has been distributed to 1 kg in first trimester and 5 kg in second and third trimester.[29]

It is inadvisable to allow pregnancy weight gain to become excessive. It may be due to excess fluid retention and could be first sign of pre-eclampsia. An average of 12.5 kg is advised. If the weight gain is less than normal, stationary or falling it may be due to intrauterine growth restriction (Table 4.2).[15,29]

Ideally weight gain should depend upon pre pregnancy BMI level.[29]
- Weight gain for a woman with normal BMI (20-26) is 11-16 kg.
- An obese woman (BMI > 30) should not gain more than 7 kg.
- Underweight woman (BMI <19) may be allowed to gain up to 18 kg.

Table 4.2: Total weight gain for single fetus.[19,20]

Fetus	3.36–3.88 kg
Placenta	0.48–0.72 kg
Amniotic fluid	0.72–0.97 kg
Uterus and breasts	2.42–2.66 kg
Blood and fluid	1.94–3.99 kg
Muscle and fat	0.48–2.91 kg
Total	9.70–14.55 kg

Edema

In the third trimester there is increase in fluid retention which results in edema of hands, ankle and feet in most women. This can reduce joint ROM and cause pressure on nerves and this can result in carpal tunnel syndrome.[12,15]

Fundal Height and the "Lie" of the Baby

Compare the gestational age and symphysio fundal height of uterus. Normal growth is 1 cm per week ± 2 cm. At 32 weeks symphysio-fundal height should be 30-34 cm. Less than 30 cm may indicate intrauterine growth retardation (IUGR) or oligohydramnios. Greater than 34 cm may indicate multiple pregnancy, polyhydramnios or macrosomia. In case of multiple pregnancies, the fundal height gets increased. In second trimester of pregnancy, the fetus will frequently change the position. By the time of 36 weeks, 93% of cases will be in cephalic position.[13,15,28]

Fetal Movements

It is noticed by the mother between 16 and 22 weeks of gestation. Fetus starts moving since 8 weeks but mother cannot feel it because; uterus is not sensitive to touch. It will be felt by the mother only when it contacts with the anterior abdominal wall. In case of subsequent pregnancy, the women will feel movements early. May be because she is already experienced this sensation before and she is aware about the sensation. Fetal movements are used to measure the baby's health. Decrease or stoppage of normal fetal movement may indicate serious complications. "Kick charts" are used to monitor the well being of baby. The mother makes note of first ten movements per day. Record the time and strength of kicking. The longer the time spans for ten movements the greater the concern.[14,15,28]

Fetal Heart Rate

It is preferable to question mother about fetal movements that she feels, rather than listen to baby's heart rate, this will be good indicator of fetal well being. It cannot be heard before 20 weeks using stethoscope. The normal rate will vary between 120 and 160 beats per minute.[15]

EXERCISE PRESCRIPTION[16,17,24,26]

Therapist must closely monitor the patient and adjust the exercise according to patient's condition.

Frequency: Minimum three times per week and preferably daily.

Intensity: Woman who used to do regular exercise before pregnancy, exercise intensity must not exceed pre-pregnancy levels. Use the talk test to monitor the exercise intensity. HR ranges related with moderate intensity exercise have also been developed for pregnant women based on age.

Time: Moderate intensity exercises minimum 15 min/day and gradually increases to at least 30 min/day (Avg-150 minutes/week).

Mode: Exercises which use large muscle groups should be prescribed. Weight bearing and non-weight bearing exercises both are safe during pregnancy, as long as she is comfortable. Non-weight bearing exercises like swimming and cycling improves physical as well as mental health and weight bearing exercises like walking, jogging and low impact aerobics improves physical fitness.

ANTENATAL PHYSIOTHERAPY FOR FIRST TRIMESTER OF PREGNANCY

In the first trimester strenuous exercise should be avoided as it may lead to miscarriages. Concentrate on improving posture, strengthening of pelvic floor, relaxation and breathing exercises.[17]

Table 4.3: Heart rate range according to age of pregnant women[17,19,20]	
Age (Years)	Heart Rate (beats/minutes)
<20	140–155
20–29	135–150
30–39	130–145
>40	125–140

Low Impact Aerobic Exercises

Depression is common among pregnant women and it is associated with increased risk of prenatal and postnatal complications. Exercise is an effective therapy for depression. According to studies, 3 months of aerobic exercise training helps to reduce the severity of symptoms of depression among pregnant women.[18,25]

Walking

It is one of the best exercises for the pregnant women. It is safe and helpful throughout the nine months and can be built into day to day schedule. Shoe with proper fitting and support must be prescribed. Studies prove that, everyday 30 minutes of walk improves birth outcome.[13,19,26]

Swimming

It is the best and safest non-weight bearing exercise which provides cardiovascular workout, helps to stretch and tone the muscles in antigravity environment, and helps to minimize joint damage and balance problems. During first trimester, minimum 20 minutes swim 3 times a week is beneficial.[13,20,26]

Stationary Bicycling

It is excellent aerobic exercise during first trimester of pregnancy and has less risk of fall than standard bicycle. It helps to avoid joint strain and easy for woman who is new to exercise.

Breathing Exercises

Breathing pattern shows mental and physical level of the woman. Breathing is slow and rhythmic when at rest and become erratic and shallow in stressful situation. She may hold her breath in this situation. Breath control will help her to know her state and also help to relax. This will help to reduce the time duration for normal vaginal delivery and also reduce the physical damage during labor. During a contraction, the aim of breathing exercise is that her thought processes are re-directed from a pain response to a learned relaxed breathing response. The woman will develop relaxed response to painful stimuli only through practice.[14-16]

Deep Breathing Exercise

Deep breathing exercise is the most efficient method of breathing during pregnancy for pregnant woman and fetus. This technique assists the women to relax, improve circulation of blood, boosts the supply of oxygen to mother and fetus both.[17-20]

- Sit comfortably with back supported in a well ventilated setting.
- Close eyes, relax shoulders, facial expression, jaw muscles and release any tension.
- First, ask her to notice natural pattern of breathing.
- Now ask her to inhale deeply and slowly through nose.
- Ask her to fill lungs and imagine breathing deeply into abdomen. During breath in, her abdomen should move forward.
- Ask her to breathe out through mouth. During breath out her abdomen should move downward.

Pelvic Floor Exercises

Pelvic floor muscle exercises must be started in the first trimester of pregnancy as a preventive strategy for urinary incontinence. It helps to prepare for childbirth and prevents uterine prolapse, urinary incontinence and haemorrhoid.[21-23,26,27]

Finding Pelvic Floor Muscles

For finding pelvic floor muscles, ask woman to trying to stop passing gas and flow of urine at the same time. By doing this, woman will feel "squeeze and lift" of pelvic floor muscles. Ask her to continue the contraction for as long as she can (upto 10 seconds) then release and relax for some seconds. Repeat this procedure as many times she can upto maximum of 10 repetitions. It helps to improve the endurance of pelvic floor muscles.[24,25]

Precautions must be taken while doing this exercise. Perform this exercise without:
- Contraction of buttocks
- Breath hold
- Squeezing legs together

Women can do this exercise during normal day to day activities. For example, while cleaning teeth. If a woman is unsure that she is exercising the right muscles, ask her to put thumb into the vagina and perform the exercises. She should feel a gentle squeeze as the pelvic floor muscle contracts. It is very important to learn the exercises properly, and therapist must check that woman is doing these exercises correctly.[26,27]

Antenatal Physiotherapy

❖ Sit comfortable. Keep feet and knees apart. Lean forward and place elbows on knees. Continue normal breathing and keep all the muscles relaxed, specially muscles of stomach, legs and buttocks.
❖ Ask her to imagine trying to pass a wind and stop passing urine at the same time. While doing this she must feel squeezing and lifting of pelvic floor muscles.

Posture Awareness

Postural awareness helps to release tension, improves blood supply and function of autonomic nervous system which in turn improves the functioning of reproductive organs, and reduces strain of muscles, joints and ligaments.[28,29]

Standing Posture

❖ Head and Neck: Head should be relaxed and balanced on the top of the spine with neck straight.
❖ Shoulders and Arms: The arms hang comfortably by sides freely without any tension. Both shoulders must be at the even height.
❖ Legs and Feet: The feet should be foot apart with the toes facing forward. Weight should be taken equally on both the feet.

Stretching Exercises

Stretching exercises are implemented with precaution. Because of hormonal changes connective tissues and supporting joint structures are at increased risk of injury from forceful stresses during pregnancy and the immediate postnatal period.[29]

❖ **Low back stretches (Cat and Camel Exercise)**
  Patient Position: Quadruped Position
  Procedure:
  - In quadruped position, relax the head and allow it to drop.
  - Round the back up towards the ceiling until the stretch is felt in the back.
  - Hold the stretch position till it feels comfortable or around 15 to 30 seconds.
  - Then return to the starting position with flat back.
  - Now sway the back by pressing abdomen toward the floor and lift buttocks toward the ceiling.
  - Hold this position for 15 to 30 seconds or till it feels comfortable.
  - Repeat 2 to 4 times.

Physiotherapy in Obstetrics

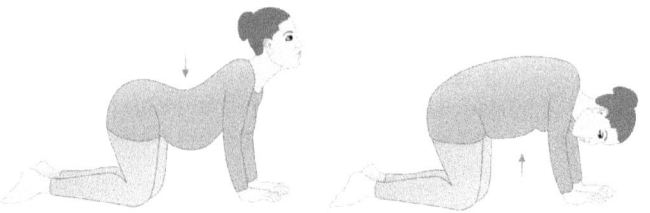

Figure 4.1: Low back stretches.

- **Backward stretch**
  Patient position: Quadruped position
  Procedure:
  - Start with the quadruped position.
  - Curl backward towards your heel till it feels comfortable at the knees.
  - Tuck the head towards the knees and keep arms extended.
  - Hold for 10 seconds and then return to the starting position.
  - Gradually work upto 10 repetitions.

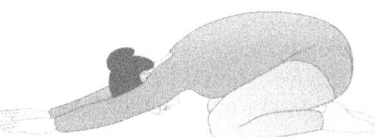

Figure 4.2: Backward stretch.

- **Backward stretch with fitness ball**
  Patient position: Stand in kneeling position and hands on the fitness ball.
  Procedure:
  - Stand in kneeling position and arms straight on the fitness ball.
  - Slowly curl backward towards heel till it feels it comfortable at the knees.
  - Hold for 10 seconds and then return to the starting position.
  - Gradually work upto 10 repetition.

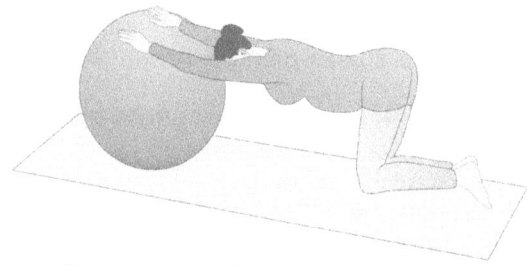

Figure 4.3: Backward stretches with fitness ball.

Antenatal Physiotherapy

- **Standing posterior pelvic tilt**
  Patient position: Standing against the wall
  Procedure:
  - Stand erect against wall with feet shoulder width apart.
  - Push the back against wall and try to minimize lumbar lordosis.
  - Hold for 10 seconds and then return to the starting position.
  - Gradually work up to 10 repetition.

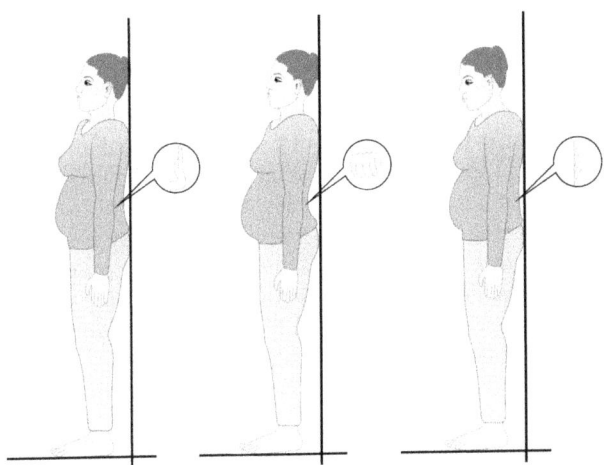

Figure 4.4: Standing pelvic tilt.

- **Trunk rotation**
  Patient position: Sitting erect with cross legs
  Procedure:
  - Sit erect on the mat and legs crossed.
  - Hold right foot with left hand.
  - Move right hand behind you and slowly turn your upper body towards right.
  - Hold till it is comfortable.
  - Return to the starting position and repeat to the other side.
  - Gradually work up to 10 repetitions on both the side.

Calf Stretching

It is very good exercise to prevent calf pain. Many pregnant women feel calf pain during pregnancy especially during second and third trimester. Regular calf stretching will help to prevent it and also helps to cure it.

Relaxation

Relaxation is necessary in pregnancy and also during the postnatal period. Generally Laura Mitchell method is taught to the women. Women can also do relaxed breathing, yoga and pranayama during antenatal period. Anulom vilom and ujjayi pranayama can be performe under the expert supervision.[30,31]

Massage

During first trimester of pregnancy, goal of massage is to provide relaxation and increase flow of circulation. Muscle tension slows lymph flow and can cause fatigue and risk of toxemia. By stimulating circulatory system, massage speeds up elimination of toxins and excess fluid, and helps to boost immunity and energy level.

Massage during first trimester should be done with precautions. The risk of miscarriage is maximum at first trimester so only trained and certified massage therapist should do the massage during first trimester. Deep abdominal massage is avoided. Massage is contraindicated in first trimester, if pregnancy is high risk pregnancy.

Yoga

Yoga is a form of exercise with breath control which helps to maintain and improve mental, physical and spiritual health. Especially in the first trimester of pregnancy, it helps in mental and physical relaxation. It should be done with care and under the guidance.
The Asanas:
- Savasana
- Katichakrasana
- Veerasana
- Dandasana
- Tadasana (The standing pose).

ANTENATAL PHYSIOTHERAPY FOR SECOND TRIMESTER OF PREGNANCY

In the second trimester, all signs of nausea disappear. Women will feel extremely well both physically and emotionally. Exercise is important to protect against strain and injury, to boost the circulation of both lymph and blood, to keep muscles toned and for sense of well being. Avoid exercising in supine or prone position after the first trimester. Continue all first trimester exercises and also add the following exercises. All the exercises must be done according to the advice of trained physiotherapist.

Back and Pelvis Care

Back and pelvis pain is frequent complain and needs extra care during and after pregnancy. This pain is due to relaxation of ligamentous structures in spine, pelvis and direct pressure caused by the gradually enlarging uterus. Change in hormone levels will cause softening of ligaments. Due to this, back and pelvic joints will not be well supported and can get strained. The baby weight and altered COG puts extra strain on these structures which can lead to back and pelvic girdle pain. The other reason for back pain is increase in lumbar lordosis due to bending forward to counterbalance the forward shift of center of gravity.

During pregnancy, recommended weight gain is 11 to 16 kg. Approximately half of this weight is gained in the abdominal area. The enlarging abdomen causes postural compensations that frequently cause back and pelvic pain. Generally LBP begins in the second trimester around 22nd weeks of pregnancy. The 50% of women, who have back pain during pregnancy, will continue to have pain even after delivery for around 1 – 3 years. PGP usually begins by the end of first trimester and peaks between the 24th and 36th gestational weeks. Usually this will resolve within 6 months after delivery but in 10% of women, the pain continues for 1 – 2 years after delivery.

- Avoid bending over low surface. Raise the surface, sit down or kneel down for any work.
- Lift equal weights in each hand while shopping or lifting during any work.
- While lifting weight, hold the object as close as possible to the body and keep back straight.
- Always lift weight by flexing knees not by stooping down.
- Sleep in a side-lying position with pillow support under the abdomen and flexed knee.
- Get in and out of bed from side.
- Back should be supported while sitting.

Exercises to Prevent and also Treat Back Pain during Pregnancy

- Practice Cat and camel exercises (Low back stretches), backward stretches.
- Practice good posture during sitting, standing, sleeping and even during work.
- Standing pelvic tilts.
- Bridging

Abdominal Exercises

As the baby grows abdominal muscles will stretch and weaken. Thus, strong abdominal muscles can also help to prevent chances of diastases recti.

- **Planks:** Planks must perform with the care. Women can perform planks only if she was exercising even before the pregnancy and only if she is comfortable in doing planks. Hold the position till the woman is comfortable then be relaxed. Never overdo it. Stop the exercise or reduce the hold timing if it feels uncomfortable. Woman can also perform side planks if she is comfortable.
- **Modified Squats:** Supported wall squatting helps to strengthen the core muscles and lower limb muscles. It also stretches the perineal area and help to push the baby during labor and delivery. If woman is planning to use squatting position for labor, that muscles must have adequate strength and endurance.

  Procedure: Ask woman to stand straight and supported against wall with feet shoulder width apart. Breathe in and raise arms straight in front of chest. Then slowly squat down towards the floor as much as she can. Breathe out as she squat down. Then slowly come back to the starting position with breathe in. Try to do two sets of 15 repetitions but start with the comfortable repetitions then progress slowly according to the woman's ability. Gradually progress to 50 – 60 seconds hold. If woman want to adopt this position during labor, it is necessary to improve endurance for the comfortable and shorter second stage of labor.
- **Side-lying SLR:** This exercise will also help to strengthen gluteus and hip abductor muscles. While performing SLR in side-lying make sure her hips are in line with the body. Perform it gently and carefully. Repeat it 10 times each side. Breathe in while lifting the leg up and breathe out while taking it down.

Drink water or stay hydrated while doing any exercises. Take sips in between the exercise. Never overdo it. Stop immediately if she feels uncomfortable or if it hurts. Do not overdo abdominal exercises as overdoing the abdominal exercises can increase the fetal blood pressure and can cause fetal tachycardia. Stop doing exercise if she feels increase in heart beat or exhausted. If woman is not exercising before the pregnancy, then start with the exercise 5 minutes a day then gradually extend the time as it is comfortable for the woman.

Antenatal Physiotherapy

Foot and Ankle Exercises[7,15]

These exercises will help to reduce or prevent pitting edema, varicose vain, cramp and improve circulation.
Knees must be relaxed for both exercises.
- Do alternate ankle plantar flexion and dorsiflexion.
- Circle both feet in each direction. (Clockwise and Anticlockwise)
- Repeat both of these exercises 30 repetitions regularly.

Many pregnant women experience calf pain, especially during night. This exercise will help to prevent calf pain and also cure it. Calf stretching, toe standing, immersion of leg in warm water and also regular calcium intake along with this exercise will be very good in case of calf pain.

Posture and Comfort Positions

Standing[18,31]
- Stand up tall and feel lower abdomen muscles.
- Shoulder must be relaxed and breathe normally.
- Body weight should be equally distributed on both the feet.

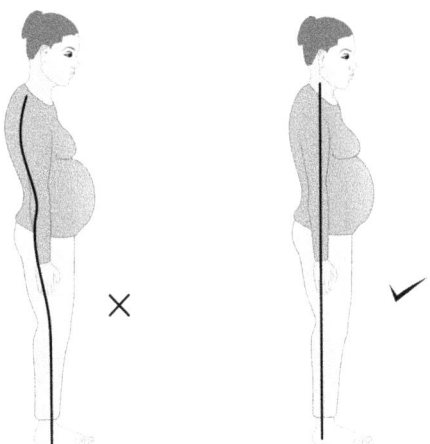

Figure 4.5: Standing posture.

Sitting[18]
- While sitting, back should be well supported and straight.
- Use a small cushion to support lumbar lordotic curve.
- Feet should be well supported on the floor or on the stool.
- Avoid crossing legs and feet as it can cause (SI) joint pain.

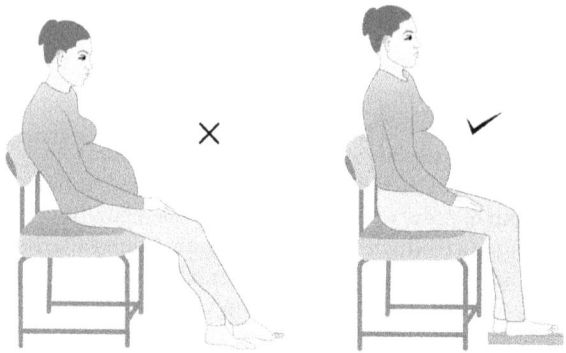

Figure 4.6: Sitting posture.

Lifting[18]

- ❖ Lifting things incorrectly can cause back problems and pain.
- ❖ For safe lifting, put one foot in front of the other with back straight and flex the knees while reaching down.
    - Keep the object as close as possible to the body.
    - Gently contract pelvic floor and abdominal muscles and keep the back straight, avoid twisting movements and breathe out while standing up.
- ❖ Avoid lifting and moving heavy objects.

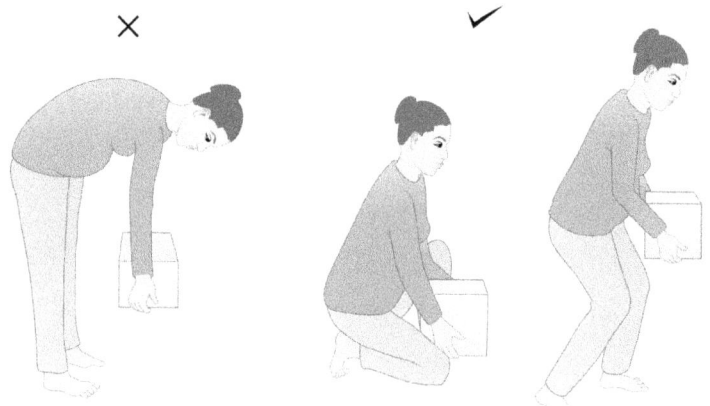

Figure 4.7: Lifting posture.

Sleeping Positions[18]

Supine lying position may be uncomfortable during pregnancy. Sleeping positions given below will make woman more comfortable.

- **Side-lying:**
  In side-lying position, use a pillow between knees and under the abdomen.

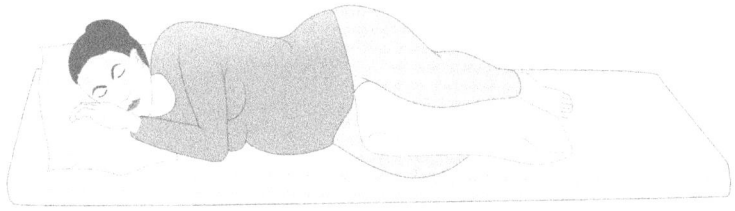

Figure 4.8: Side-lying posture.

- **In three quarters lying:**
  In this position, use pillow to support upper leg.

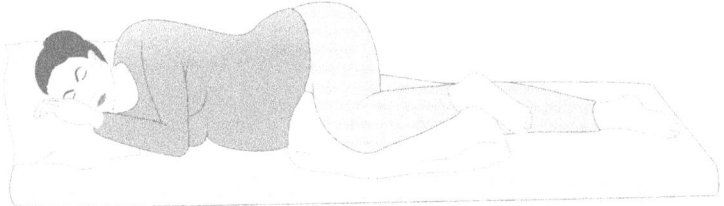

Figure 4.9: Three quarters lying posture.

- **On your back:**
  Supine lying is not recommended. Put pillows to raise and support the head, shoulder and upper back. Use pillow under the knees for more comfort.

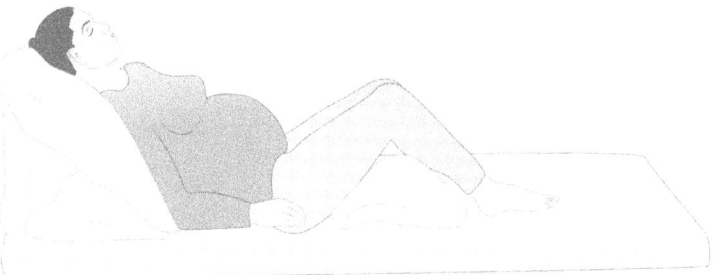

Figure 4.10: Supine lying posture.

Getting On and Off the Bed

- Flex the knees.
- Gently contract abdominal and pelvic floor muscles and turn to the side with a back straight.
- Swing lower limb over the side of the bed and use upper limb to push the body into a sitting position.
- Do the reverse to get on the bed.

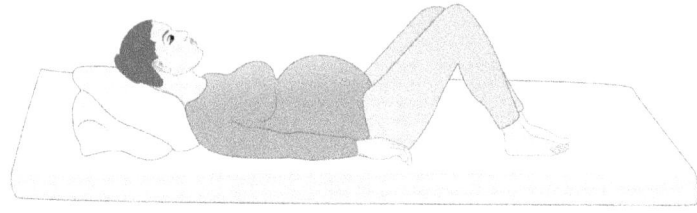

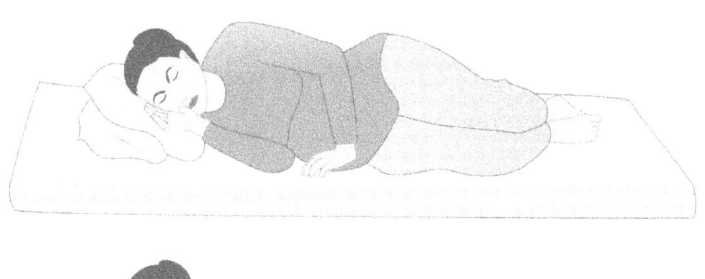

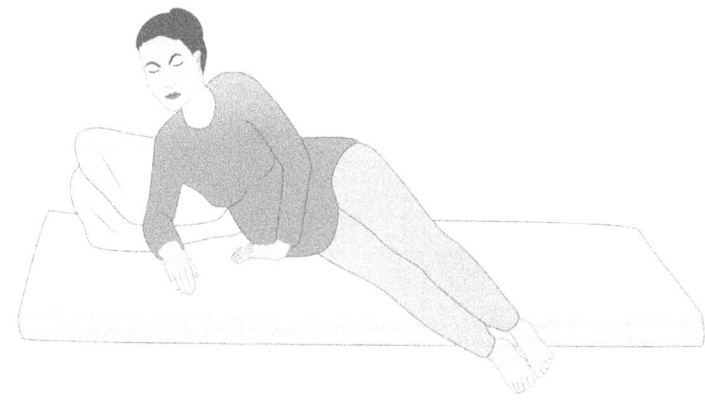

Figure 4.11: Getting off and on the bed.

Shopping

Shopping bags should be divided equally in both the hands. This will help to avoid pelvic girdle pain and also help to maintain balance.[31]

Hydrotherapy

The hydrotherapy leads to decrease in systolic and diastolic blood pressure. These changes will lead to decrease in ADH, aldosterone and plasma rennin activity. The change in blood volume causes decrease in vital capacity, ventilatory capacity and expiratory reserve volume. According to studies, hydrotherapy will minimize the risk of joint injuries and there are no any adverse effects on the fetus.

Massage

During the second trimester, weight of the baby will increase and that can cause muscle soreness. The belly becomes more apparent with the growth of baby. The highest risk of miscarriage has passed. Massage is used to relieve muscle spasms, soften the connective tissues, relieving back pain and leg cramps.

Yoga

In the second trimester, it helps to stabilize the pelvis, strengthen the core and lower limb muscles and also induce mental relaxation.
The Asanas:
- Tadasana (The Standing pose)
- Trikonasana (The triangle pose)
- Veerasana
- Katichakrasana (Pelvic rotations to sides)

ANTENATAL PHYSIOTHERAPY FOR THIRD TRIMESTER OF PREGNANCY

In the third trimester, women feel the extra weight. Exercise plays an important role in reducing the edema and correcting postural imbalance. The relaxation and breathing technique are the best exercises.

Massage

Perineal Massage

Perineum will get stretch and it gets strained frequently during the labor. Episiotomy is indicated in case of failure of perineum to stretch or chances of bad tear. Perineal massage is effective to avoid episiotomy. Research shows that perineum massage daily for 5-10 minutes, especially in age group of 30 years and above in the last 6 weeks of pregnancy and in second stage of labor will prevent second or third degree perineal tear or the chances of episiotomy and instrumental delivery.[30,31]

Woman can herself or her partner can perform this massage technique. Ask her to sit in squatting and lean back in a well supported position and then perform the massage.

Technique

- Before starting massage, make sure that bladder is empty. Then take a warm bath. It will help to stretch the tissue and relax it.
- Take any natural oil and massage perineum and lower vaginal wall. Place about 5 cm of either the thumbs or index fingers inside vagina and perform "U" type movement upward and to the sides of the vaginal wall with downward pressure to stretch the perineum to the maximum from side to side until she feels burning and tingling sensation which is similar to the feeling when baby's head begins to crown. Maintain this stretch for 30-60 seconds then release. Ask woman to be relax, take regular breath and not to hold breath during massage. This will help her to learn relaxation during delivery.
- Conscious relaxation of pelvic floor muscles during labor will help to prevent tissue damage. Initially it may be difficult to relax pelvic muscles consciously. But the moment when she experiences tingling or burning sensation during massage, try to relax pelvic floor muscles.

Yoga

If can be continued if comfortable. The main goal of yoga in third trimester is relaxation.

The Asanas:
- Tadasana (The standing pose)
- Modified savasana.

GUIDELINES FOR MANAGING THE PREGNANT WOMEN[31]

- Do not exceed 5 minutes of supine positioning after the first trimester of pregnancy to avoid vena cava compression by the uterus. Compression of the vena cava also occurs with motionless standing. For supine exercise, place a small wedge or rolled towel under the right hip to lessen the effects of uterine compression on abdominal vessels

and improve cardiac output. The wedge turns the patient slightly toward the left. This modification is also helpful during examination and treatment when the patient is positioned supine.
- To avoid the effects of orthostatic hypotension always rise slowly when moving from lying position or sitting to standing positions.
- Avoid Valsalva maneuver because this may lead to undesirable downward forces on the uterus and pelvic floor. Breath-holding causes stress to the cardiovascular system in terms of blood pressure and heart rate.
- Take break frequently for fluid replenishment. The risk of dehydration during exercise is increased in pregnancy.
- Encourage complete bladder emptying before exercise. A full bladder places increased stress on an already weakened pelvic floor.
- Include warm-up and cool-down for at least 5 minutes.
- Modify or discontinue any exercise that causes pain.
- Advice woman to wear supportive footwear to reduce musculo-skeletal stresses.
- Avoid single leg weight bearing activities, such as standing leg kicks. It can cause loss of balance, sacroiliac or pubic symphysis discomfort.
- Avoid full squats, cross-steps, rapid direction changes and ballistic exercise.

Most modalities are contraindicated in pregnancy. Superficial heat or ice may be beneficial along with manual techniques prenatally to relieve pain and spasm and improve circulation.

Recommendations for Fitness Exercises

- For strength and cardiopulmonary benefits, it is strongly recommended for all women to participate in regular mild to moderate exercise for around 15 to 30 minutes/session, most days of the week are recommended. Exercise program should not exceed pre pregnancy exercise level.
- There are no data that pregnant women need to decrease their intensity of exercise or lower their target heart rates, but due to decreased oxygen supply during pregnancy, according to their tolerance level they should modify exercise intensity. Conventional, age-based target heart rate may be too aggressive for the average pregnant women. Use of the Borg scale of perceived exertion is more appropriate in this population, with exertion between 12 and 14 suggested during pregnancy. A woman should stop exercising when fatigued and never exercise to exhaustion.

- During pregnancy, woman must avoid contact sports, high altitude (>6000 ft) activities, activities with risk of abdominal trauma or falling and scuba diving. During scuba diving, fetus is at increased risk of decompression sickness.
- Proper nutrition, adequate fluid intake, and appropriate clothing for heat dissipation are important.
- Continuation of pre-pregnancy exercises during the postpartum period should be gradual.

SACROILIAC JOINT PAIN/POSTERIOR PELVIS PAIN/PELVIC GIRDLE PAIN[19]

SI joint pain can occur at one or both sides with or without radiating pain to the buttock and posterior thigh but not to the leg and foot.

SI joint is stable joint and permits very little movement. Pain may begin at any time during antenatal or postnatal period but commonly begins at the 18th weeks of pregnancy and may increase as the pregnancy progresses. According to one study, there is four times greater incidence of posterior pelvic pain than LBP in pregnant woman.

The SI joint is stable through two mechanisms:
- The rough, groove like connecting surfaces of the sacrum and ilium interlock with each other and helps to stabilize the joint.
- SI joint is strengthened by ligaments and muscles. These core muscles such as transverse abdominis and multifidus acts as active stabilizers by actively contracting to create a compressive force over the SI joint and gripping the joint together. They act as a natural corset by providing compression around the lower back and pelvis.

SI joint pain arises when stability of SI joint is compromised.

Causes of SI Joint Pain

During pregnancy, mechanisms stabilizing SI joint is affected. This instability, allows increased joint ROM and stress the SI joint.
- Hormones released during pregnancy, relax the ligaments to allow the pelvis to enlarge in preparation for childbirth.
- Weakness and stretching of core muscles due to enlargement of uterus.
- Weight of fetus and altered walking pattern can cause mechanical strain on SI joints and may result in inflammation and pain.

Symptoms

❖ Deep and aching pain around the SI joint which get worsen with activities like prolonged sitting, standing walking, stair climbing, resting on one leg, getting in and out of low chair, rolling and twisting in bed and lifting weight.
❖ Radiating pain to groin and thighs but not to the feet.
❖ Pain gets reduced in lying position.
❖ If there is inflammation and arthritis in the SI joint, woman may experience stiffness and burning sensation in the pelvis.

Management

In case of pregnancy related SI joint dysfunction, initially focus should be on core stability of trunk and pelvic girdle. Sacroiliac belt can be prescribed especially during walking to reinforce the core stability exercises and give quick pain relief. The manual techniques like mobilization, mulligan mobilization, muscle energy techniques and myofascial release can be used to correct any movement dysfunction.

Modifications of daily activities:
❖ Single leg weight bearing should be avoided.
❖ Excessive lower limb abduction should be avoided.
❖ Sitting on very soft surface should be avoided.
❖ Getting into a car is done by sitting down first then pivoting both legs and trunk into the car. Avoid lower limb abduction during getting in and out from the car.
❖ During a sidelying, place a pillow between the knees and under the abdomen.
❖ Avoid climbing more than one step at a time.
❖ Avoid crossing the legs when sitting.

Modifications of exercises:
❖ Avoid exercises that require single leg standing.
❖ Avoid exercises that require abduction or hyperextension.
❖ Teach the patient to activate the transverse abdominals and pelvic floor when transferring from one position to another to stabilize the pelvis.

EFFECT OF SUPINE LYING DURING PREGNANCY

In normal healthy pregnancy, if woman is comfortable, she can adopt any position but there are some physiological changes of supine lying in late pregnancy.

Cardiovascular Symptoms

During pregnancy, supine lying is not advisable during and after the second trimester. To reduce the risk of low blood pressure (supine hypotensive syndrome), supine lying is not preferable position. There are many physiological especially cardiovascular changes occur during pregnancy. As the pregnancy progresses, there are increase in cardiac output, stroke volume and heart rate so that the oxygen demand of mother and fetus can be fulfilled. These cardiac parameters decreases when woman change position from side-lying to supine in late pregnancy. There is almost complete occlusion of inferior vena cava and lateral displacement of subrenal aorta in supine lying during late pregnancy because of compression by uterus. It is known as aortocaval compression syndrome. Cardiac output, stroke volume and heart rate are greatest in left side-lying position. Therefore left side-lying is the most preferable position as early as 20 weeks of gestation.

Respiratory Symptoms

During third trimester, supine lying causes narrowing of upper respiratory airways. Due to this dyspnea and snoring are most common complains and woman is not comfortable in supine. But this will not affect the fetal circulation or growth.

STUDY QUESTIONS

1. Explain about back and pelvic care during pregnancy.
2. Technique and importance of perineal massage in antenatal period.
3. Importance of prenatal exercises and benefits of exercise during pregnancy.
4. Explain about relaxation techniques in antenatal period.
5. Antenatal back care program.
6. Role of exercises towards easy labor.
7. Weight gain in pregnancy.
8. Plan an antenatal class.
9. Massage in labor.
10. Discuss the basic principles of exercise program and explain the need for them during pregnancy. Identify harmful exercise that should be discussed with the client.
11. The patient presented with the following complains:
    o History of missed periods for the last 2 months.
    o Nausea 2 weeks after missed period.
    o Breast heaviness

The patient had regular menstrual cycles until 2 months ago. Two weeks after her missed menses, the patient started experiencing nausea in early morning, breast heaviness and laziness. She suspected the possibility of pregnancy. She performed a home pregnancy test which was positive; therefore she came for medical advice. Advice her about the same.

REFERENCES

1. NICE–National Institute for Health and Care Excellence, 2014.
2. Britnell SJ, Cole JV, Isherwood L. Postural Health in Women: The Role of Physiotherapy, Canada. Canadian Physiotherapy Association. 2005; 159:493-500.
3. Antenatal Exercises and Advice. NHS Trust–The Pennine Acute Hospitals, 2013.
4. Antenatal Exercise. Department of Health and the Hong Kong Physiotherapy Association. 2013. pp. 65-8.
5. Pelvic Floor Exercise for Women, Janseen-Cilag Ltd. London, 2008.
6. Artal R, Clapp JF, Vigil DV. Exercise during Pregnancy, American College of Sports Medicine.
7. Obstetric Physiotherapy Service, Health Improvement Service, Antenatal Exercises, HSC–Northern Health and Social Care Trust.
8. Artal R, Toole MO. Guidelines of the American College of Obstetricians and Gynecologists for Exercise during Pregnancy and the Postpartum Period, Australia. 2015;8:6-12.
9. Breathing and Relaxation Exercises and Tips for Working with Pain in Labour. Falkirk Print Works, 2016.
10. Casagrande D, Gugala Z, Clark SM. Low back pain and pelvic girdle pain in pregnancy. The American Academy of Orthopedic Surgeons. 2015;23(9):539-49.
11. Vince C, Nwuga B. Pregnancy and back pain among upper class Nigerian Women. The Australian Journal of Physiotherapy. 1982;28(4):8-11.
12. Bell BB, Dooley MM P. Exercise in Pregnancy, Royal College of Obstetricians and Gynecologists. 2006.
13. Antenatal Exercises, New Mowasat Hospital, Canada.
14. Hammer RL, Perkins J, Perr R. Exercise during the childbearing year. The Journal of Perinatal Education. 2000;9,(1).
15. Polden M, Mantle J. et al. Physiotherapy in Obstetrics and Gynecology. Elsevier Limited, 2004.
16. Pelvic floor Exercises. International Uro-gynecological Association, 2011.
17. Madhuri GB. Physiotherapy for Obstetrics and Gynecological Conditions. Jaypee Publications, 2007.
18. G A Dumas, J G Raid, M P Griffin. Exercise, posture and back pain during pregnancy. Clinical biomechanics. Elsevier Ltd. 1995:10;104-9.

19. Kisner C, Colby LA. Therapeutic Exercise–Foundations and Techniques. Philadelphia, Margaret Biblis Publishers. 2007,(5).
20. M. Sarfraz et al. Role of physical therapy in antenatal care as perceived by the clients - a cross sectional survey on pregnant females attending antenetal OPD. Pakistan Journal of Medicine and Dentistry. 2013:1(01); 34-6.
21. Abrecque M, Eason E, Marcoux S. Randomized controlled trial of prevention of perineal trauma by perineal massage during pregnancy. American Journal of Obstetrics and Gynecology. 1999;180(3):593-600.
22. Eason E, Preventing Perineal Trauma During Childbirth: A Systemic Review. Elsevier Inc, Canada. 2000;93(3):464-71.
23. Colson JHC, Collison FC. Progressive Exercise Therapy, 4th edition. John Wright and Sons Ltd, USA.
24. Thompson WR. ACSM's Guidelines for Exercise Testing and Prescription, 8th edition, Philadelphia: Lippincott Williams & Wilkins. 2010.
25. Robledo AF. Colonia, et al, Aerobic exercise training during pregnancy reduces depressive symptoms in nulliparous women: a randomized trial, Australian Physiotherapy Association. Journal of Physiotherapy. 2012;58: 9-15.
26. Advice for Physiotherapists and Other Health Professionals. Association of Chartered Physiotherapists in Women's Health, 2016.
27. Urinary incontinence in women: Management. NICE Guidelines, 2013.
28. Fairley DH. Obstetrics and Gynecology, 2nd edition. Blackwell Publishing, London. 2004.
29. DC Dutta, Konar H. DC Dutta's Textbook of Obstetrics, 8th edition. Jaypee Brothers Medical Publishers, 2015.
30. Shipman MK, Bonyface DR, Tefft ME, et al. Antenatal perineal massage and subsequent perineal outcomes: A randomized controlled trial. British Journal of Obstetrics and Gynecology. 1997;104:787-91.
31. Downie PA, Boardman S. Cash's Textbook of General Medicine and Surgical Conditions for Physiotherapists, 2nd edition. Jaypee Brothers. 131-61.

CHAPTER 5

Physiotherapy during Labor

Chapter Outline
- Stages of Labor
- Comfort Measures to Manage Pain and Suffering in Labor

INTRODUCTION

The exact mechanism of initiation of labor is not known. Labor is divided into three stages, each stage contains specific events. The primary symptom of labor is regular and strong involuntary contractions of the smooth muscles of the uterus. True labor produces effacement and dilation. These changes are palpable in the cervix.[1]

Definition of Labor: Sequential events in the genital organs to expel the fetus, placenta and membranes out of the womb through the vagina into the outer world are called labor.

Effacement: It is the thinning of the cervix before the onset of labor from a thickness of 5 cm to the piece of paper.[1]

Dilation: It is the opening of the cervix from the diameter of a fingertip to approximately 10 cm.[1]

STAGES OF LABOR

Labor—Stage 1[1-3]

This is the longest stage of labor. Some women experience initial cervical dilation and effacement before the true labor. By the end of this stage, the cervix is fully dilated and baby is about to be delivered. Stage 1 of labor is divided into **three phases:**

a. **Cervical dilation phase:** Also known as early labor phase. It will last approximately 8 to 12 hours. The cervix dilates from 0 to 3 cm. Mild and irregular but progressive uterine contractions occur from the top down, causing the cervix to open and pushing the fetus downward.
b. **Middle phase:** Also known as active labor phase. It will last approximately 3 to 5 hours. Contractions will last about 4560 seconds with 3-5 minutes rest in between. The cervix dilates from 4 to 7 cm. Contractions are stronger, longer and more regular. It is good time to start breathing techniques and relaxation exercises between contractions. Ask woman to drink plenty of water and urinate periodically. Massage her lower back and abdomen. Remind her to change positions frequently or walk. Provide distractions from labor such as music, playing simple game like cards, painting etc.
c. **Transition phase:** It is a labor milestone, exhausting and emotionally draining. The cervix dilates from 8 to 10 cm and dilation is complete. Uterine contractions are very stronger, close together and can overlap. This phase can last from 30 minutes to 2 hours. Contractions will last for 60-90 seconds with a 30 second-2 minutes rest in between. Women's legs may tremble and have cramps. Women may lose the ability to concentrate, become impatient, tired, angry, frustrated and irritable. She may also experience nausea, vomiting, chills, hot flashes or gas. Some women start to have doubt about their ability to deliver baby. Transition is a psychological as well as physical state.

Labor—Stage 2[1]

Stage 2 begins with the complete dilatation of the cervix, involves pushing and expulsion of the fetus. Due to complete dilatation of the cervix, the membrane rupture and good amount of amniotic fluid escape. Volume of uterine cavity will reduce. Intra-abdominal pressure is the primary force expelling the fetus. It is produced by voluntary contraction of the abdominal muscles and diaphragm. Relaxation and stretching of the pelvic floor during stage 2 are also necessary for successful vaginal delivery. Uterine contractions may last as long as 90 seconds during this stage.

Fetal descent: Position changes (cardinal movements) by the fetus allow it to pass through the pelvis and be born. The position changes (Fig. 5.1) are described as:
a. **Engagement:** The greatest transverse diameter of the fetal head passes through the pelvic inlet, the superior opening of the minor pelvis.
b. **Descent:** Downward progression of the fetus will continue.

c. **Flexion:** The fetal chin is brought closer to its thorax. This occurs when the descending head meets resistance from the walls and floor of the pelvis and the cervix.
d. **Internal rotation:** When the fetal head reaches the level of the ischial spines, the fetus turns its occiput toward the mother's symphysis pubis.
e. **Extension:** The flexed fetal head reaches the vulva. The fetus extends its head; bring the base of the occiput in direct contact with the inferior margin of the maternal symphysis pubis. This phase ends when the fetal head is delivered.
f. **External rotation:** To allow the fetal shoulders to pass through the pelvis, the fetus rotates its occiput towards the mother's sacrum.
g. **Expulsion:** The fetal anterior shoulder passes under the symphysis pubis, and the rest of the body follows.

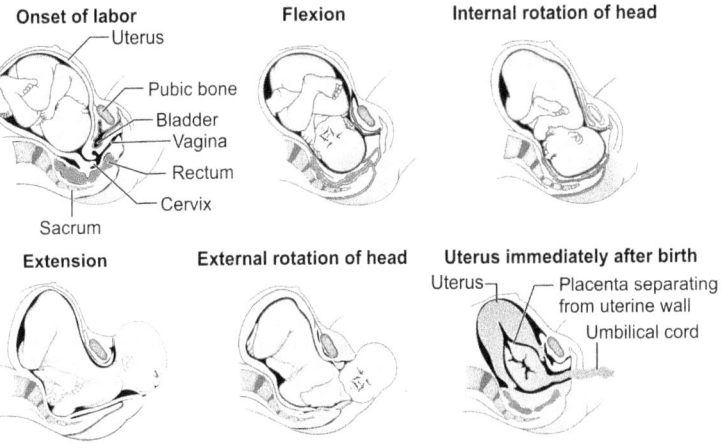

Figure 5.1: Fetal descent positions.

Labor—Stage 3[1]

a. **Placental separation (expulsion of the placenta):** After delivery, the uterus continues to contract and shrink, causing the placenta to detach and be expelled. It is expelled out by voluntary contraction of the abdominal muscles or by manual procedures.

The uterus decreases in size 5-30 minutes after the baby is delivered. The placenta detaches from the uterine wall, blood vessels are constricted, and bleeding slows. A hematoma forms over the uterine placental site to prevent further significant blood loss. Mild bleeding will be continued for 3 to 6 weeks after delivery.

b. **Uterine involution:** For 3 to 6 weeks after delivery the uterus continues to contract and decrease in size. The uterus always remains slightly enlarged over its pre pregnant size.

COMFORT MEASURES TO MANAGE PAIN AND SUFFERING IN LABOR

Breathing[4,1]

Breathing techniques during labor will help to reduce muscle tension and bring enough oxygen to both pregnant women and baby.
- Slow, deep diaphragmatic breathing is the most efficient method during labor.
- Teach the woman to relax the abdomen during inspiration so that it feels as though the abdominal cavity is "filling up."
- During exhalation, the abdominal cavity becomes smaller. Active contraction of the abdominal muscles is not necessary with relaxed breathing.
- To prevent hyperventilation, emphasize a slow rate of breathing.
- Advice the woman to decrease the intensity of the breathing if she experiences dizziness or feels tingling in the lips and fingers.
- In the first stage, as labor progresses natural free respiration which will increase in rate and depth.

Different Authors have their recommendations for breathing during labor. They are given in the Table 5.1.

Relaxation

Visual Imagery

Use instrumental music and verbal guidance. Instruct the woman to concentrate on a relaxing image such as the beach, mountains, or a favorite vacation spot. She must focus on the same image throughout the pregnancy so that the image can be called up to the conscious level when recognizing the need to relax during labor.[1,3,4]

Relaxation and Breathing[1]

First Stage

- The contractions of the uterus become stronger, longer, and closer as the labor progresses. Relaxation during the contractions becomes more difficult. Provide assistance to the woman in relaxation.

Physiotherapy during Labor

Table 5.1: Recommendations for breathing during Labor

Author	First Stage	Transitional Stage	Second Stage
Dick and Read (1942)	Natural free respiration which increases in rate and depth as labour progresses. 24 – 28 full breaths / minute. Abdominal and upper thoracic respiration.	Breathing will be at its fastest and deepest rate.	Train women to hold breathe to push. After each expulsive effort, 2 – 3 full deep breaths were taken. Rapid shallow panting for delivery.
Williams and Booth (1985)	"Easy breathing" Little slower and deeper than usual–12 beats / minute. "Lighter breathing" – Upper chest rises and falls. 24 – 28 beats / minute.	Breathing to prevent pushing: "fairly deep" breathing to move the diaphragm up and down, with a sharp blow out through relaxed lips.	1 or 2 deep breaths in and out, then hold the breath making the diaphragm "piston" goes down. Repeat when breath runs out, after a gulp of air.

- Ensure that the woman has emotional support from the Mother, Husband, family member, or special friend to provide encouragement and make her comfortable.
- Relax in comfortable positions like walking, lying on pillows and pelvic rocking.
- Breathe slowly with each contraction. Use the visual imagery and relax with each contraction. Focus attention on a specific visual object. Women can do singing or talking during each contraction to prevent breath holding and encourage slow breathing.
- Near the end of the first stage, during transition, there is often an urge to push. But this is not the appropriate time to push so to overcome this urge, teach the woman to use quick blowing techniques using the cheeks, not the abdominal muscles.
- Massage to areas that hurt such as the lower back. It may help the woman to distract the focus from the contractions.
- Apply heat or cold for local symptoms. Wipe the face with a wet and clean cloth.

Second Stage

Once dilation of the cervix has occurred, the woman may become active in the birth process by assisting the uterus during a contraction in pushing the baby down the birth canal. Teach her the following techniques:
- While pushing down, breath in, contract the abdominal wall, and slowly breathe out. This will cause increased pressure within the abdomen along with relaxation of the pelvic floor.
- If woman holds her breath, there will be increased tension and resistance in the pelvic floor.
- Maintain relaxation in the extremities, especially the legs and perineum. Keep the face and jaw relaxed. This will helps to maintain maximum efficiency.
- Try to perform total body relaxation between contractions.
- As the baby is delivered, just "let go" and breathe rapidly with short gaps or sigh to relax the pelvic floor as it stretches.

Transcutaneous Electrical Nerve Stimulation

Many medical professionals are not aware about the effects of TENS during labor. It has no side effects on mother or baby. Specialized TENS machine appropriate for pregnancy and birth is used. TENS unit designed for other uses are not appropriate for labor. TENS is more effective when used with other coping strategies like relaxation, positioning and/or massage. 1 in 5 women in the UK try TENS for their labor. Research shows that TENS is most effective when it is used in early labor and then continued throughout labor.[3]

Electrode Placement

- Electrodes need to be positioned over the nerve pathways which transmit pain from uterus and cervix.
- One pair of electrode each side of T10 – L1.
- Another pair of electrode each side of S2 – S4.

Parameters

- Frequency: 80 – 120 Hz
- Pulse duration – 150 μs
- Intensity: It must be enough to block the pain. As the labor progresses, gradually increase the intensity. The current must feel strong but comfortable. It is usually operated by the woman herself.

Specialized TENS Machine

It has booster control with two outputs:
- Continuous output of high frequency and high intensity – used during contractions
- Burst output of low frequency and low intensity – used between contractions

Mechanism of Pain Control

TENS relieves pain by the pain gait control theory. It also releases natural pain killers like endorphin which helps to relieve or reduce the pain sensation during labor.

Benefits of TENS during Labor

- It has no side effect on mother or baby.
- It is a form of non-invasive pain relief.
- It allows mother to be free and change position easily as needed.
- It can apply at home during early labor.
- Easy to use.

Positions in Labor

Changing of position and stay upright during labor has many benefits to both baby and pregnant woman compared to supine lying. Research shows following disadvantages of supine lying position in labor:[5]
- More painful and less effective contractions.
- Longer labor.
- Reduced blood flow to fetus.
- Narrower passage through the pelvis for fetal descend.

Positions for First Stage of Labor

Proper positions during the first stage of labor provide pain relief, help woman to cope with pain and reduce the use of epidural analgesia and the duration of first stage of labor.[6]

For Resting

- **Side-lying**: Place pillow between knees for relaxation and comfort.[5]

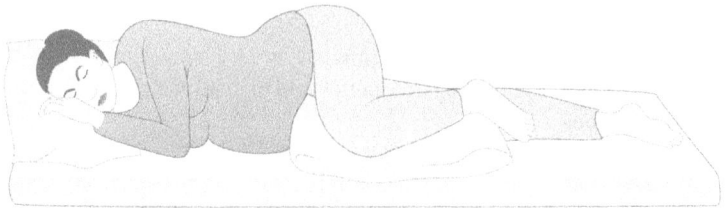

Figure 5.2: Side-lying position.

- **Semisitting in bed**:[5]

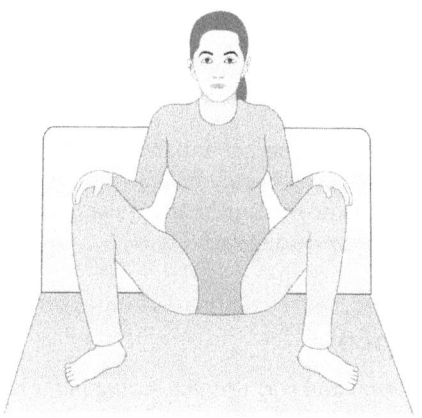

Figure 5.3: Semisitting position.

- **Sitting with one foot up**: This position helps to change the shape and enlarge the pelvis, which helps in fetal descend.[5,6]

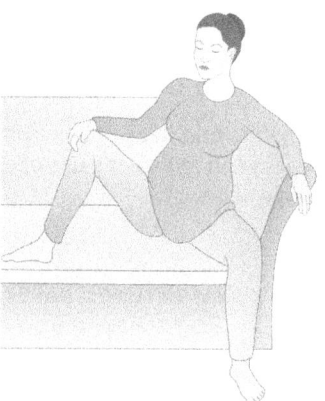

Figure 5.4: Sitting position with one foot up.

Physiotherapy during Labor

- **Rocking, rhythmic motion:** Some woman feels better using a rocking and swaying movements during first stage of labor.[5,9]

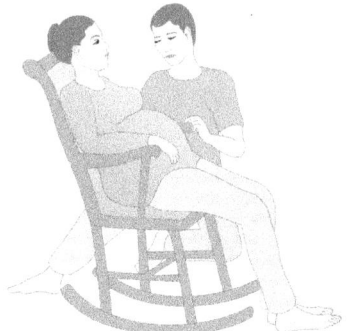

Figure 5.5: Rocking chair.

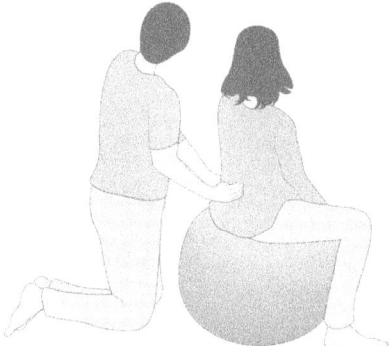

Figure 5.6: Sway on ball.

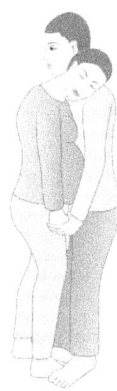 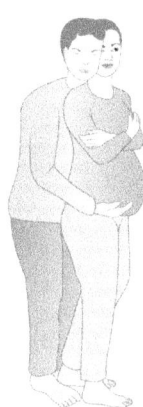

Figure 5.7: Slow dancing.   **Figure 5.8:** Dance with belly lift.

❖ **Activity:** Walking, climbing stairs, lunges. These activity helps in fetal descend and helps fetus to rotate into position for birth. In early stage of labor, advice to be active but do not exhaust. Walking is more effective during active labor and transitions to encourage the cervix to open and to reduce the duration of labor.

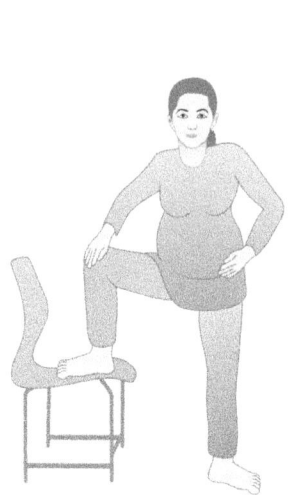

Figure 5.9: Lunge.

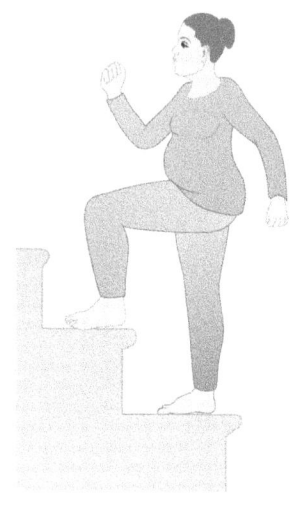

Figure 5.10: Stair climbing.

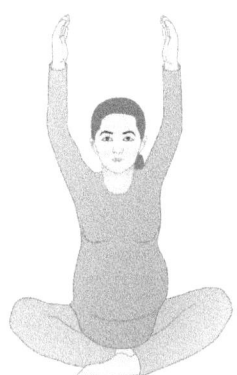

Figure 5.11: Tailor stretching.

Positions for Back Labor (Lower back pain and irregular contractions in lower back) and when labor is progressing slowly:

Many women with back labor find it most relaxing to lean forward during contractions.[5,7-10]

Physiotherapy during Labor

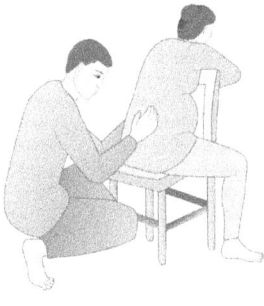

Figure 5.12: Straddle a chair.

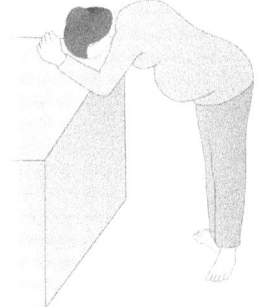

Figure 5.13: Leaning against wall.

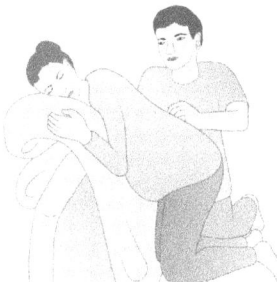

Figure 5.14: Raise the end of the hospital bed, and then kneel on bed with arms resting on top of the bed.

Kneeling

Kneeling helps to relieve back pain. Back massage can be done easily in this position. It will make easier to sway side to side, rocking movement or do pelvic tilts to increase comfort. Advice woman to use knee pad while kneeling or kneel on something soft to protect knee joint.[5,10]

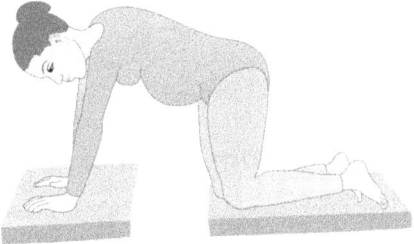

Figure 5.15: Kneeling.

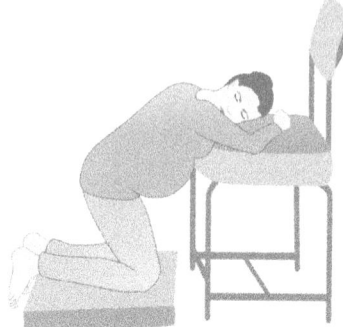

Figure 5.16: Chair supported kneeling.

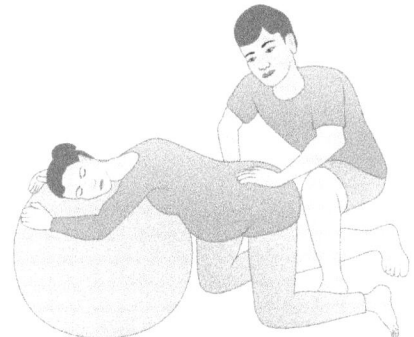

Figure 5.17: Over birth ball.

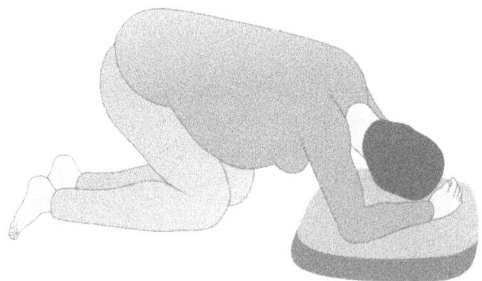

Figure 5.18: Knee chest.

Positions for Second Stage of Labor

Upright position is comfortable in second stage of labor which includes sitting (>45 degrees from the horizontal), squatting, kneeling and quadruped position. Recumbent positions include supine, lateral and semi-recumbent positions with wedge.[6,7,10]

"Standard" Positions

- **Semi-sitting position**: In this position, use pillows under knees, arms and back. During contractions ask woman to wrap hands around knee and pull knees towards shoulders. This is common position in hospital setting and important for midwives as it provides good view and easy access to perineum.[5,10]

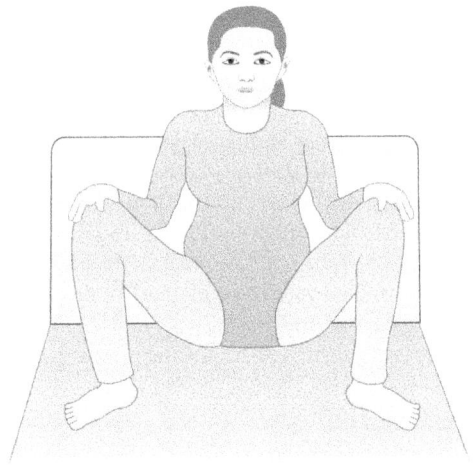

Figure 5.19: Semi sitting position.

- **Side-lying**: Back should be curved and upper leg should be supported her partner. This position is good for fast second stage. Shorten et al. stated that it is more comfortable position for woman and also helps to protect and prevent tearing of perineum.[5,10]

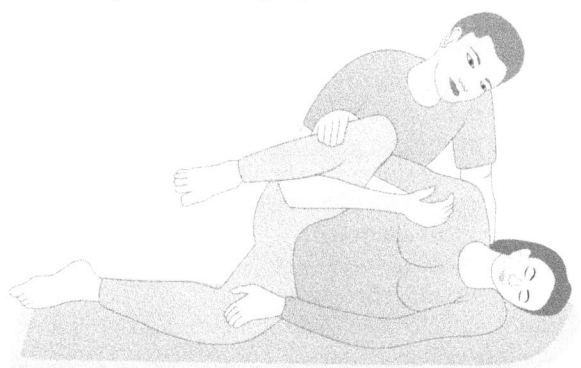

Figure 5.20: Side-lying position.

Squatting using a birth chair has been reported as a predisposing factor for third and fourth degree tears. Woman should be encouraged, helped and also physically and emotionally supported to move and adopt whatever position is most comfortable for her throughout the labor.[6,10]

Avoid Perineal Tearing During Stage 2

Stage 2 of labor involves pushing and expulsion of the fetus. So there are more chances of tearing of perineum. With the help of some strategies we can try to avoid tearing of perineum.
- Perineum massage during antenatal period. (For detail methodology check Chapter no 4 Antenatal physiotherapy)
- Perineum massage during stage 2 of labor.
- Stretching of pelvic floor muscles during stage 2 of labor.
- Water birth
- Birthing positions like squatting and quadruped position can reduce pressure on the perineum.
- Warm compresses on the bottom during pushing.

STUDY QUESTIONS

1. Describe about the stages of labor and explain in detail about resting positions in first stage of labor.
2. Relaxation techniques in labor pain.
3. "Relaxation exercises"—list the type of this in physiotherapy. Explain its role in pregnancy and labor.
4. Identify the breathing exercise to be used in labor. Describe the physiological effects of the same.
5. Role of physiotherapy modalities in conducting pain free labor.
6. 32 year old female 7 months pregnant, complaining of right sacroiliac joint pain. Advice her about some self help measures to manage pain. She is also curious to know about labor positions to adopt during labor to avoid exacerbating the pain in her joints.
7. True contractions characterized by all except:
   a. Occur at regular intervals
   b. **Pain stop with sedation**
   c. Pain felt in back and abdomen
   d. Intervals get gradually smaller.
8. False contractions (Braxton Hicks) characterized by all except:
   a. Occur at irregular intervals
   b. Intensity doesn't change

c. **Cervix dilate**
d. Pain primarily in lower abdomen.

REFERENCES

1. Kisner C, Colby LA. Therapeutic Exercise–Foundations and Techniques, 5th edition. Philadelphia, Margaret Biblis Publishers, 2007.
2. Claire M. Andrews et al. Maternal position, labor and comfort. Applied Nursing Research. 1990;3(1):7–13.
3. Madhuri GB. Physiotherapy for Obstetrics and Gynecological Conditions. Jaypee Publications, 2007.
4. Breathing and Relaxation. Wellington – Dufferin – Guelph Public Health.
5. Positions in Labor. NHS Trust–Wrightington Wigan and Leigh. 2014; Obs 041:1–9.
6. Munro J, Jokinen M. Positions for Labor and Birth. The Royal College of Midwives, 2012.
7. Gupta JK, Hofmeyr GJ, Smyth R. Position in the Second Stage of Labour for Women without Epidural Anaesthesia. The Cochrane Collaboration, John Wiley and Sons Ltd. 2007, Issue 4.
8. Lawrence A, Lewis L, Hofmeyr GJ. Maternal Positions and Mobility during First Stage Labor. The Cochrane Collaboration, John Wiley and Sons Ltd. 2009, Issue 4.
9. Scott Brittnel, et al. Postural health in women: The role of physiotherapy. Journal of Obstetrics and Gynaecology. Canada, May 2005.
10. Dutta SC, Konar H. DC Dutta's Textbook of Obstetrics. Jaypee Brothers Medical Publishers, 8th edition, 2015.

CHAPTER 6

Postnatal Physiotherapy

> **Chapter Outline**
> - The Effect of Exercise on Recovery from Labor and Delivery
> - Physiotherapy Management Guidelines
> - Ergonomic Principles
> - Postural Exercises
> - Immediate Postnatal Problems
> - Long-Term Postnatal Problems
> - Abdominal Muscle Exercises
> - Training of Pelvic Movements
> - Pelvic Floor Awareness, Training and Strengthening
> - Warning Signs to Slow Down
> - Advice on Activities Related to Baby
> - General Postnatal Physiotherapy Management Protocol

INTRODUCTION

First and the most important goal of postnatal physiotherapy is to restore pelvic floor muscles and core abdominal muscles as these muscles give support to spine, pelvic girdle and also helps to prevent complications like urinary incontinence. There are less chances of developing postnatal depression if woman become active after delivery as soon as possible. Return to exercise must be gradual. Ligaments laxity will be present up to 5 months after the birth so care must be taken and do not resume high impact activity too soon.[1-3]

The speed of return to normal pre-pregnancy routine depends on the duration and difficulty of delivery. In case of long labor with complications or instrumental delivery, woman need more recovery time. Many physiological and psychological changes take place even after the delivery. Because of hormonal changes, ligament and muscle laxity is common and it is the common cause of injury in postnatal period. Immediate return to

physical training program is difficult. Body is undergoing many changes at this time including:[3,6]
- Decrease in uterus size
- Weight loss
- Hormonal changes
- Changes in breasts
- Tightening of muscles stretched in pregnancy
- Tightening of joints
- Decrease in blood volume
- Drop in heart rate.

THE EFFECT OF EXERCISE ON RECOVERY FROM LABOR AND DELIVERY

Continuation of physical exercise is very important in postnatal period. It will help:[3,7]
- Improve muscle strength and endurance
- To relax and improve muscle tone which get imbalanced during pregnancy and delivery.
- To reduce the risk of postnatal depression and improve psychological health.

PHYSIOTHERAPY MANAGEMENT GUIDELINES (TABLE 6.1)

Ask woman to start gentle exercises as soon as she can, within 24 hours of the birth will achieve best results. Ask woman to do gentle exercises and that should not be harmful. Very quickly it will help her to get back to fitness.[4]

General Advice[2,7,8]

- *Rest*: Advice her to take rest whenever she can. Sleep when baby is sleeping, Take offers of help.
- *Hygiene*:
  - Keep stitches clean.
  - Watch for infection, bad smell, pain, fever or shivering.
- *Urine*: Drink at least two liters of water per day. Do pelvic floor exercises to prevent leakage of urine.
- *Bowel movements*:
  - Remember the importance of good diet to prevent constipation.
  - Hold a clean sanitary towel against stitches when going to toilet to support the stitches.

Table 6.1: Physiotherapy management guidelines for postnatal women.[7]

	Goal	Plan of treatment
1	To develop awareness and control of posture.	Posture awareness training. Stretching, training and strengthening of postural muscles.
2	To learn safe body mechanics.	Teach body mechanics during ADLs, with infant and during infant care activities.
3	Develop upper extremity strength it will be necessary for infant care.	Resistive exercises to appropriate muscles.
4	Develop awareness and control of the pelvic floor muscles.	Awareness of pelvic floor muscle contraction and relaxation. Train and strengthen the pelvic floor muscles.
5	Maintain abdominal function and prevent or correct diastasis recti.	Monitor diastasis recti. Diastasis recti exercise. Abdominal strengthening exercises with diastasis recti protection.
6	Promote or maintain cardiovascular fitness.	Safe progression of aerobic exercises.

- ❖ Wear loose and light cloths.
- ❖ Wear supportive training shoes.
- ❖ Wear well supporting sports, maternity bra.
- ❖ Do not exercise when feeling unwell.
- ❖ Avoid overheating: Exercises in controlled climate or air conditioned environment during hot or humid days.
- ❖ Stay hydrated.
- ❖ Exercise within the limit of talk test.
- ❖ Warm up and cool down before and after the aerobic workout.
- ❖ Avoid the prone knee-chest position for at least 6 weeks postpartum because of the risk of air embolism.

ERGONOMIC PRINCIPLES[9,13]

It is necessary to educate woman about proper ergonomic principles as wrong posture can cause or even exaggerate back pain, knee pain, pelvic girdle pain, etc. During postnatal period, body needs to be kept in correct posture during rest and during activities. It will help the spine to re-align and get back to the normal curvature.

Sitting

- Thighs should be fully supported.
- Sitting surface should not extend from popliteal fossa otherwise it can cause impingement.
- Feet should be flat and fully supported on the stable base of support.
- Body weight should be evenly distributed over both the buttocks.
- Woman should sit on the cushion if she is having sore perineum or hemorrhoids.
- Sitting surface should be depressible to allow pressure distribution.
- Trunk should be fully supported and maintain natural curvatures of spine.

Standing

- Feet should be hip distance apart hips should be slightly laterally rotated (following true line of femur).
- Weight should be evenly distributed over both the feet.
- Soft knees. Full extension of knee but do not ask her to lock them back.
- Shoulders relaxed.
- Arms held loosely at the side.
- Maintain normal curvature of side of the body.
- Maintain normal curvature of spine.

Lying

- Body should be fully supported. Use pillows for relaxation at head, knees and low back.
- Legs should not be crossed.

Kneeling

- Sustained, isometric trunk flexion or rotation should be avoided.
- Try to keep movement within the sagittal plane.
- Activities should be performed at proper height.

POSTURAL EXERCISES

During pregnancy, postural muscles get stressed due to height and weight of the growing fetus. Center of gravity shifts upward and forward. Spine shifts to compensate and maintain stability. After delivery activities of caring and holding the baby put stress on postural muscles. To balance these postural muscles stretching and strengthening of specific muscles is recommended stretching and strengthening exercises must be done with precaution because connective tissue and supporting joint structures are at increased risk of injury from forceful stresses due to hormonal changes during pregnancy (Table 6.2).[7,8]

IMMEDIATE POSTNATAL PROBLEMS

Perineal Dysfunction/Pain

Perineal pain is the common symptom in postnatal phase especially for those who are recovering from episiotomy. Perineum is the area of skin between the vagina and the anus. If the perineum has been damaged or repaired, it can cause pain, requiring analgesia and woman may prefer to sit on rubber ring. Visible problems include bruising, edema, labial tears, hematoma, tight stitches, infection and breakdown of suturing. Vaginal hematoma will not be visible but it will be painful.[9]

Treatment

Pelvic floor muscle exercises
It is the most important technique for the perineal pain relief. It must be started as soon as possible. Most of the woman avoids it due to pain and swelling. But gentle and rhythmic contractions boost the healing process and reduce swelling and so the pain. Woman have to do the slow repeated contraction and relaxation of the pelvic floor muscles. This pumping action assist in venous and lymphatic drainage and that will help to remove traumatic exudates, relieve stiffness and pain and helps

Table 6.2 Stretching and strengthening of specific muscles.[7]	
Stretching (with precautions)	*Strengthening (low intensity)*
Upper neck extensors and scalene	Upper neck flexors, lower neck and upper thoracic extensors
Scapular protractors	Scapular retractors and depressors
Shoulder internal rotators, and levator scapulae	Shoulder external rotators
Low back extensors	Trunk flexors (abdominals), particularly lower abdominals
Hip flexors (iliopsoas), adductors, and hamstrings	Hip extensors
Ankle plantarflexors	Knee extensors
	Ankle dorsiflexors

to restore function. According to some theories it stimulates the pain gate mechanism and produce endogenous opioids. Maximum pain is felt with the first contraction and pain and edema reduces as patient continues the exercise. Woman must be comfortable while performing these exercises. The position will be according to symptoms and depends on the comfort level of woman. Initially most comfortable position, like lying on bed is preferable. (For detail methodology of exercise refer Chapter 4). Doing pelvic floor exercises every time she feeds her baby will help her to regain pelvic floor muscle strength.[1,4,6,7,9]

Cryotherapy:[9]
Cryotherapy will reduce pain, swelling and gives soothing effect.
Crushed Ice:
Woman can apply crushed ice wrapped in disposable gauze, towel or plastic bag (to avoid drips) to the affected area for 10 to 15 minutes. A Plastic acts as an insulator and therefore effectiveness is reduced. Ice packs specially designed for perineum are also available.
Ice cube massage:
Woman can use ice cube held in a tissue. It will give excellent pain relief.

Warm baths:[9]
It promotes good hygiene. Warm water can also be poured over perineum. This ease the burning sensation some woman experience when urinating, if they have sustained lacerations.

Warm sitz bath:
Warm sitz baths can also be given for 20 minutes two times a day. In sitz bath only hips and buttocks are immersed in water. This will also ease discomfort, reduce pain and swelling.

Ultrasound:[9]
According to studies, ultrasound increases the tissue temperature, which will increase the blood flow and tissue repair. It should be started as soon as possible after delivery.

Patient Position: Crook lying or Side-lying

Dosage: Pulsed ultrasound, 3 MHz, 0.5 W/cm^2, 2 times per day until the patient is able to do all the functional activities without pain.

It is not necessary to change the dosage if there is improvement in pain and decrease in swelling. If woman have more intense pain due to direct contact of ultrasound head, a condom can be used as a water bag. This will also make the application of ultrasound more comfortable for the patient.

Pulsed SWD/Pulsed Electromagnetic Energy (PEME):[9]
It helps to relieve pain, bruising, large hemorrhoids, post cesarean birth hematomas and inflamed or infected wound.

Dosage: 40 – 65 pulses with repetation of 10 – 220 pulses/second, twice a day, initially for 5 minutes then progress to 20 minutes.

With the all these treatments woman must be aware about some little self help techniques that will also help her to be comfortable like, avoid tight cloths that can rub and irritate the area and slow healing. If she is feeling perineal pain while passing the bowel, advice to drink lots of fluids and eat more fibers.

Diastasis Recti (Fig. 6.1)

The Greek word "Diastasis" means "separation" and "Recti" refers to the "Rectus Abdominis" muscle. Diastasis recti is the common condition of pregnancy and postpartum characterized by separation of the rectus abdominis muscles in the midline at the linea alba. The etiology of this separation is unknown. The continuity and integrity of the abdominal musculature are disrupted. Any separation more than 2 cm or two finger width is considered significant. A study, done by Bursch, found a significant diastasis in 62.5% of postpartum women tested within 92 hours of delivery. The rate of diastasis recti is higher in non-exercising woman than in exercising woman.[7,8]

Due to hormonal effects on the connective tissue and the biomechanical changes of pregnancy, diastasis recti may occur anytime during last half

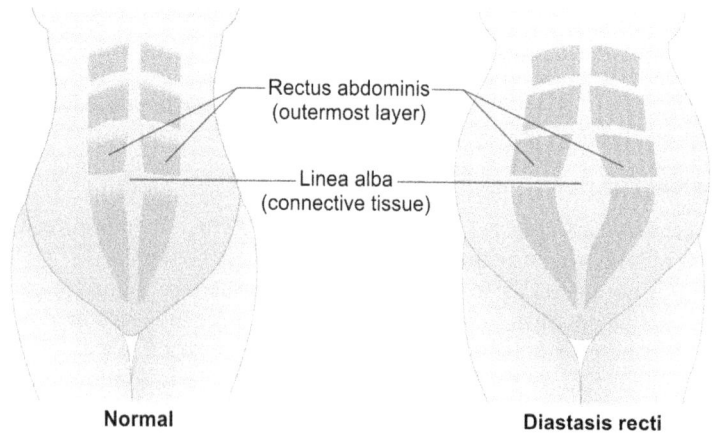

Figure 6.1: Diastasis recti.

of pregnancy but it is most commonly seen after pregnancy. It may also develop during labor, especially with excessive breath-holding during the second stage. It causes no discomfort. It can occur above, below, or at the level of the umbilicus but it is less common below the umbilicus. It appears to be less common in women with good abdominal tone before pregnancy. Routine assessment for this condition is highly recommended and can easily be done with abdominal strength testing.[7]

Significance[7]

Diastasis recti can produce low back pain, constipation and urinary incontinence. Constipation and lifting heavy weights even lifting newborn baby, can strain the muscles and can make condition worst.

- **Functional limitations:** Inability to perform independent supine to sitting transitions because of extreme loss of the mechanical alignment and function of the rectus muscle. It can also affect the normal breathing pattern of the woman.
- **Herniation:** Severe cases of diastasis recti (longer than 10 cm and wider than 2 cm) can progress to herniation of the abdominal viscera through the separation at the linea alba. It requires surgical repair. Rehabilitation following this type of repair may include components of C-section rehabilitation, with specific precautions and input from the referring surgeon.

Examination for the Presence of Diastasis Recti[7]

Test all pregnant women for the presence of diastasis recti before starting any abdominal exercises. This test should be repeated throughout the pregnancy and appropriate modifications made to existing exercises. Instruct patients to perform a self-test on or after the third postpartum day. Until 3 days after delivery, the abdominal musculature has inadequate tone for valid test results.

Patient position: Hook-lying.

Procedure: Have the woman slowly raise her head and shoulders off the floor reaching her hands toward the knees, until the spines of the scapulae is off the floor. Place the fingers of one hand horizontally across the midline of the abdomen at the umbilicus. In case of separation, the fingers will sink into the gap between the rectus muscles. Note the number of fingers that can be placed between the muscles. Diastasis recti can also present as a longitudinal bulge along the midline. Test above, below, or at the level of the umbilicus as this condition can occur at all three areas.[7,9]

Management

Teach the woman to perform the corrective exercise for diastasis recti. Be careful while prescribing exercises. Crunches, sit ups, pushups, press ups and front planks can worsen the diastasis recti. Due to the angle of attachment of the obliques into the linea alba, there is a possibility that trunk rotation exercises can worsen the separation. Do not start training until diastasis has been diagnosed adequetly:

- ❖ Minor diastesis recti (±5 cm in length and 1 cm width) will generally correct itself naturally once woman start stimulating abdominal muscles.
- ❖ Mild diastesis recti (upto 10 cm in length and 2 cm width) will not be able to be fully corrected. Abdominal exercises may help to prevent any health issues from arising.
- ❖ Severe diastesis recti (longer than 10 cm and wider than 2 cm) will not be corrected by exercise and needs surgery. Increased pressure and tension in the abdomen cannot be absorbed by abdominal muscles, even when these muscles are highly trained. Umbilical hernia can occur at this stage.

Once the correction has been obtained, strengthening of the obliques muscles and more advanced abdominal work can be done.

Corrective Exercises for Diastasis Recti

i. Head lift[7] (Fig. 6.2)

Patient position: Crook lying with hands crossed over midline.

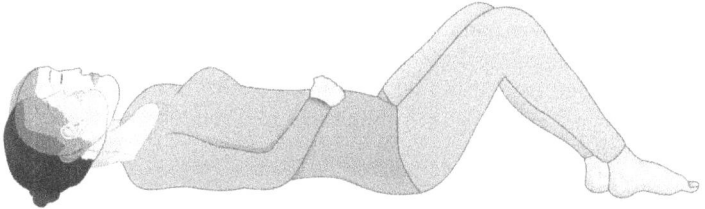

Figure 6.2: Head lift.

Procedure: Ask the woman to breathe out and lift head off the floor or until the point just before a bulge appears. At the same time, ask her to gently approximate hands to the rectus muscles toward midline. Then ask her to lower the head slowly, breath in and relax. This exercise gives special attention to the rectus abdominis muscle. Some women may not be able to reach over their abdomen. In this case, ask her to wrap towel around the trunk at the level of the separation. It will help to provide support and approximation of separated muscle.

ii. **Head lift with pelvic tilt[7,9] (Fig. 6.3)**
   Patient position: Hook-lying with her hands crossed over midline.

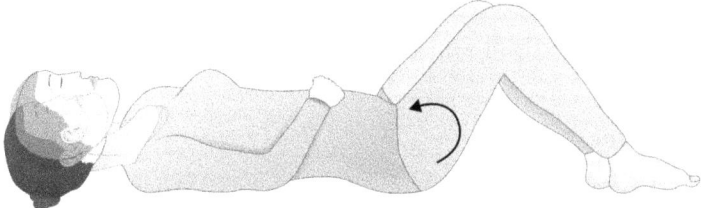

Figure 6.3: Head lift with posterior pelvic tilt to correct diastesis recti.

Procedure: Ask the woman to slowly lift her head off the floor. Approximate the rectus muscles and perform posterior pelvic tilt, then slowly lower the head and relax. To minimize intra-abdominal pressure, all abdominal contractions should be performed with breathing out.

Carefully designed pilates exercise program can also help to correct the diastesis recti. Best time to start core muscle strengthening is before the woman gets pregnant, it can prevent the complications like diastesis recti.

Tupler Technique

Tupler technique is the six weeks exercise program for diastesis recti which contains four steps and woman must follow all the four steps to achieve good results.

- **Step one:** Exercise (abdominal contractions and head lifts)
- **Step two:** Splinting the separated muscles
- **Step three:** Strengthening and learning the use of transverse muscle. (Hold transverse abdominis muscle "in" during sneezing, coughing, pick up baby etc.)
- **Step 4:** Getting up and down correctly. (Use of arms as an assistant while getting up and down).

Postural Back Pain

Back pain usually occurs due to postural changes during pregnancy, weak abdominal muscles, and increased laxity of ligaments. Study done by Ostgaard and Anderson in 1992, they found that 67% of women had back pain directly after delivery and 37% still had it even after 18 months. They compare these data with the general population and concluded that pregnancy was the cause of the back pain of the women studied.[7,9]

Characteristics

The symptoms of low back pain usually get worst with muscle fatigue or as the day progresses. Back pain is usually relieved with rest or position change. Physically fit women generally have less back pain during pregnancy.[7]

Treatment

Initially LBP can be relieved with lumbar support belt to support weak abdominal muscles, core muscle stabilization and strengthening exercises, proper body mechanics, postural and occupational instructions. Specific mobilization techniques for the sacroiliac, lumbar or lumbosacral regions can also be useful.[7,9]

Pain in Epidural Region

It can be due to presence of tiny hematoma. Hot pack or Ice pack can be used to relieve pain but proper guidance should be given about the use of both.[9]

Thoracic Pain

It can relieved by postural education, active exercises, hot pack or ice pack.[9]

Coccydynia

Coccydynia may be due to damaged ligaments, with or without displacement of the coccyx, or aggravation of previous injury. Labor is the most common cause of coccydynia. The coccyx and sacrum becomes more flexible at the end of third trimester and thus give way to the baby during labor. Sometimes a coccyx can fracture during second stage of labor and it will prevent woman to do functional activity in the early postpartum period and interfere with the mother baby bonding process. Oral analgesia may be ineffective and functional activities become intolerably painful, especially in sitting positions.

Treatment: Ultrasound, ice pack or hot pack, gentle mobilization techniques, TENS and frequent gluteal contractions can be given for pain relief. Advice to sit on the cushion or pillow as it will help to relieve pressure on the ischial tuberosity and thigh. Prone lying is the most comfortable position in this condition.[9]

Symphysis Pubis Pain[9]

Symphysis pubis pain can occur during antenatal period or after traumatic delivery. It can be gradual or sudden and give rise to disabling pain to the woman. It can be distributed to the pubic area, groin, inner thigh and suprapubic areas and accompanied by SI joint pain, low back pain or both. Sometimes clicking or grinding sound may be audible and felt by the woman. It may be unilateral or bilateral. The symptoms are aggravated by walking, turning in bed, ascending or descending stairs, weight bearing activities or any activity related to hip abduction and unilateral standing.

Treatment

Minimize weight bearing stresses until the symptoms get resolved. Mobilization should be gradual. Spinal and pelvic stability exercises can be prescribed with gradual progression. Avoid weight bearing, hip abduction, one leg standing, twisting movements and lifting. Give postural advice for functional activities to avoid aggravation of condition. Ultrasound, rest and ice pack can speed up the healing process, reduce edema and so relieves pain.

"Afterpains"

Afterpains is the name given to contractions that occur after labor. Women experience postpartum lower abdominal pains, it is known as 'afterpains' which is probably uterine in origin. These cramps are caused by contraction of uterus as it shrinks back to its pre-pregnancy state. These cramps also help to reduce postpartum blood loss. This process is known as 'involution'. Afterpains is usually mild in primiparous women. Cramping is most intense during first and second postpartum day and gradually decreases on the third day. It will take six weeks or longer for uterus to return to its pre-pregnancy state. Breastfeeding can increase these cramping because baby's sucking triggers the release of oxytocin which causes contractions.[9]

Treatment

Sleep, oral analgesics, position change, passing urine, resting in prone lying with pillow under abdomen, gentle lower abdominal massage and TENS over the T10 – L1 and S2 – S4 (nerve roots innervating uterus and perineum) can help to reduce after pains. Relaxation and breathing techniques used during labor assist in its management.

If the cramping does not stop even after few days or pain becomes unbearable, it could be the sign of infection.

Varicose Veins

Most women experience varicose veins after the delivery. Some may experience pain along the length of the long saphenous vein. It will improve following delivery, generally within three to four months after the delivery but sometimes it takes longer. In multiparus women, once veins have become varicose they will never recover completely. Woman may also develop spider veins during pregnancy. Woman will not be as active as she would normally be before pregnancy.[9]

Treatment

- Fast and frequent ankle toe movements, at least 30 repetitions at a time will prevent statis.
- Elevate leg whenever possible, use pillow below the feet while in lying position.
- Do not cross legs or ankles while sitting.
- Walking can also helps to improve circulation and minimize the symptoms of varicose veins.
- Do not sit or stand for long periods without taking breaks.
- Wear compression stockings. It helps to prevent swelling and may keep varicose veins from getting worse.

Edema[9,13]

There is massive dieresis following delivery of baby but still it can take several days or weeks for the fluid retention of pregnancy to be reversed.

Treatment

- Eat food rich in potassium as it helps to alleviate swelling.
- Stay away from processed food as it contains potassium causing bloat.
- Reduce the intake of salt.
- Consume more fluid. Drinking excess fluid will signal the body to flush out the fluids. It will help to relieve edema.
- Anti-embolic support stockings can be used for severely edematous legs.
- Rest legs in elevation. Feed baby with her legs raised. While lying down place the feet in elevation above the heart level. It will improve circulation and reduce swelling.
- Ask her to do vigorous foot and ankle exercises.
- Foot and leg massage starting from bottom and massaging upwards.
- Avoid crossing legs and standing for long period.

Superficial Vein Thrombosis[9]

Woman may complain tenderness over a palpable, superficial vein. There may be redness of the overlying skin and often associated with varicose veins.

Treatment

Be active and exercise lower limbs frequently. Use anti-embolic stockings if comfortable until the condition subsides.

Deep Vein Thrombosis

Woman will complain of pain and discomfort in calf or thigh. Swelling may be present if the vein is occluded. Homan's sign (calf pain with ankle dorsiflexion and knee extension) may be positive. Any woman with these signs should be immediately referred for medical intervention to avoid the danger of thromboembolism.[9]

Treatment

Anticoagulant therapy, anti-embolic stocking and vigorous ankle toe movements is helpful to treat this condition. If DVT is in calf, encourage woman to be mobile. Woman suffering from this condition should avoid pressure on the popliteal fossa and while sitting, legs should be elevated. If DVT is in the ilio femoral region, the woman has to take rest until the swelling subsides. Ankle toe movements, leg elevation, quadriceps and gluteal muscle contractions, hip and knee flexion and extension is helpful to improve blood circulation. Perform these exercises vigorously until the woman is able to mobilize normally.[9]

Breast Engorgement

Breast engorgement means breasts are painful, swollen and hard due to overfull of milk. Expression of milk using breast pump or hand is also very painful. This is the condition if mother makes more milk than baby uses. It can be experienced in early purperium.[9]

Treatment

Initially give ultrasound to the periphery of the breast then move towards the nipple. Warm compresses, gentle massage, crushed ice pack can be useful to relieve pain and encourage blood flow. Treatment with the pulsed electromagnetic energy is less painful as it is non-contact method.[9]

Massage: The aim of massage in breast engorgement is to reduce pain and congestion and increase circulation.

Patient position: Side-lying. Small tray is placed beneath the breast.

Technique:
- Hot water bath (10 minutes) is given to the breast prior to massage.
- Oil is used as a lubricant.
- Gentle stroking and kneading maneuvers are used from the chest wall towards the nipple 3 to 4 times.
- After this friction may be given carefully and gently over nodules.
- Repeat stroking and kneading techniques.
- Remove oil.
- Repeat hot water bath
- This technique can also be used to increase the flow of milk. But for this purpose, contrast bath is used instead of hot water bath and massage is given more vigorously.

Sore and Cracked Nipples

Sore and cracked nipples lead to discontinue breastfeeding during the immediate postpartum period. Symptoms are directly related to the position of the baby on the breast. The baby should be correctly attached and facing the mother's body with neck slightly extended, mouth well open with lower lip curled down and the nipple extending as far back as the soft palate. There should be no friction of the tongue or gum on the nipple and no in and out movement of the breast in the baby's mouth. Baby's sucking should not give any trauma or soreness to the nipple. Mother may lean forward to acquire the most comfortable position for the baby.[9]

LONG-TERM POSTNATAL PROBLEMS

Stress Incontinence

Pelvic floor muscle strengthening can help to cure stress incontinence. It must be prescribed and revised regularly according to the woman's condition. Exercise should be progressed through number of repetitions and the duration of contraction. Advice women to perform pelvic floor exercise while feeding the baby and counter brace pelvic floor muscles during activities like coughing, sneezing, laughing, blowing nose etc. If she is unable to perform or maintain contractions for more than 3 seconds, it indicates chances of denervation of pelvic floor muscles. In this case, electrical stimulation can be used. In case of urinary frequency and urgency, perform strong pelvic floor contractions to inhibit detrusor muscle activity.[9]

Carpal Tunnel Syndrom[9]

It can occur during pregnancy and usually resolves shortly after delivery. It will not cure completely until the woman is breastfeeding. Improvement will start approximately 14 days after the beginning of weaning.

Treatment

Exercise, elevation, positioning, ultrasound, ice etc can be used to treat carpal tunnel syndrome.

ABDOMINAL MUSCLE EXERCISES

During pregnancy the abdominals will extremely overstretched.

Leg Sliding[7]

Patient position: Hook lying with posterior pelvic tilt.
Procedure: Hold the posterior pelvic tilt and slide one foot along the floor until the leg is straight or to the point at which she is unable to maintain the posterior pelvic tilt. Breathe in during this movement. Then slowly slide the leg back to the starting position and breathe out. Repeat same with the other leg.

Trunk Curls[7,10]

Patient position: Crook lying.
Procedure: Curl-downs and curl-ups are very good abdominal exercises for rectus abdominis strengthening. Ask woman to protect the linea alba with crossed hands while performing trunk curls. Lift head, chest, and shoulders slightly off the bed (45 degrees). Breath in during lifting and breath out when return to starting position. Perform diagonal curls to strengthen the oblique muscles. While curling up and down, ask the woman to lift one shoulder towards the opposite knee and also protect the linea alba with crossed hands.

Bicycle in Supine[7]

Patient Position: Supine lying.
Procedure: Flex and extend the lower extremities in an alternating pattern as if cycling. Woman will feel more resistance, if she will increase the arc

of cycling movement. To avoid back strain, the woman must keep back flat against the floor and control the arc of cycling pattern.

TRAINING OF PELVIC MOVEMENTS

These exercises are helpful in cases of[7]:
- Postural back pain.
- Beneficial for improving proprioceptive awareness.
- Beneficial for improving lumbar, pelvic and hip mobility.

Pelvic Clock[7,10,11] **(Fig. 6.4)**

Patient position: Crook lying with feet shoulder width apart.

Procedure: Ask the woman to visualize the clock on her lower abdomen. The umbilicus is 12 o'clock and the pubic symphysis is 6 o'clock.

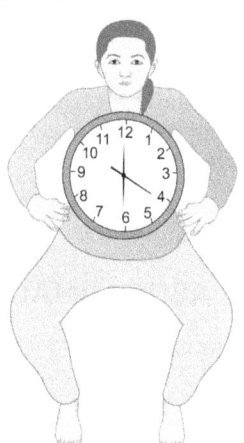

Figure 6.4: Pelvic clock.

- 12 o'clock: Slowly draw in abdominal muscles towards spine and roll pelvis towards head and flatten the back on the mat. This puts pelvis in "Posterior pelvic tilt".
- 6 o'clock: Drop pelvis towards feet. The abdominal muscles will relax and back should be arch off the mat slightly. This puts pelvis in "Anterior pelvic tilt".
- 3 o'clock: Drop left hip bone downward towards the mat and right hip bone should lift towards the ceiling.
  Be careful not to hike hip towards the shoulder. (Weight shifted to left hip).
- 9 o'clock: Drop right hip bone downwards towards the mat and left hip bone should lift towards the ceiling. Be careful not to hike hip towards the shoulder. (Weight shifted to right hip).

Then move clockwise from 12-3 to 6-9 and then back to 12 o'clock. Continue relaxed breathing throughout the exercise and do not force any part of the movement. If she has difficulty with the motion, make the clock smaller until coordination improves.

PELVIC FLOOR AWARENESS, TRAINING AND STRENGTHENING[7,11,12]

Begin pelvic floor exercise training with an empty bladder. Gravity assisted positioning may be indicated initially for some women with extreme weakness and proprioceptive deficits. As strength and awareness improves positional changes are introduced (supine, side-lying, quadruped, sitting, standing position).

Contract–Relax

Instruct the woman to tighten the pelvic floor muscles as if attempting to stop urine flow or hold the gas. Hold for 3 to 5 seconds and relax for at least the same length of time. Repeat up to 10 times.

Quick Contractions

Perform quick and repeated contractions of the pelvic floor muscles. Advice to maintain normal breathing rate and keep accessory muscles relaxed. Perform 15 to 20 repetitions per set.

"Elevator" Exercise

Ask the woman to imagine as if she is in an elevator. As the elevator goes up to the next floor, woman has to contract the pelvic floor muscles a little more. As strength and awareness improves add more "floors" to the contraction. Then ask the woman to relax the muscles gradually, as if the elevator is going down one floor at a time. This component requires an eccentric contraction of pelvic floor muscles.

Pelvic Floor Relaxation

Instruct the woman to contract the pelvic floor same as in the strengthening exercise. Then voluntarily release and relax pelvic floor muscles. Pelvic floor relaxation should link with effective breathing and relaxation of the facial muscles. During pelvic floor relaxation, ask the woman to concentrate on a slow, deep breathing and allow the pelvic floor to relax completely. Chronic inability to relax the pelvic floor muscles may lead to impairments such as hypertonus, pain with intercourse, or voiding dysfunction. If woman is having pelvic pain syndromes, increase the rest time between pelvic floor contractions.

Opening Up the Hip Rotators (Supine Butterfly Pose) (Fig. 6.5)

This is the relaxation exercise which will relax pelvic floor as well as gives mental relaxation also.
- ❖ Ask woman to lie down on a comfortable surface.
- ❖ Place sole of the feet together and open up hips.
- ❖ Abduct shoulder at 90 degrees.

- ❖ Take a deep breath in focusing on relaxing pelvic floor muscles.
- ❖ Exhale slowly while maintaining focus on pelvic floor muscles.

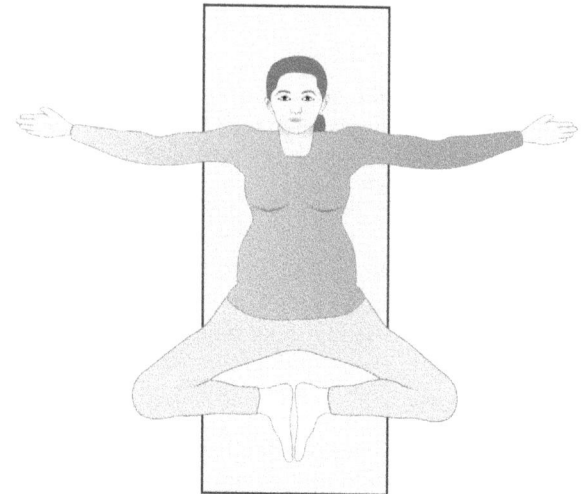

Figure 6.5: Opening up the hip rotators: Relaxation of pelvic floor muscles.

If it is difficult to open up hips, place a pillow under upper thighs and lower buttocks. Do this relaxation exercise for 10 – 15 minutes. Feel relaxed pelvic floor muscles as you deeply breathe in.

WARNING SIGNS TO SLOW DOWN[5,7]

Ask women not to overexert. Body gives warning signs if she is exercising too hard and these signs may include:
- ❖ Increased fatigue
- ❖ Muscle aches and pains
- ❖ Colour changes of lochia to bright red.
- ❖ Heavier lochia flow.
- ❖ Lochia starts flowing again after it has stopped.

ADVICE ON ACTIVITIES RELATED TO BABY[13]

Position while Feeding

- ❖ Sit on the chair with back supported. Support foot on the stool.
- ❖ Sitting tailor position may be used with the back support.
- ❖ Side-lying on bed.

Bathing or Changing

- Bath time should be fun for both mother and baby.
- Use suitable and an easily accessible height. Do not stoop. Kneel down instead of stooping.

Carrying

- Hold baby close to the body. This is important for security and well being of both mother and baby.
- Holding the baby on one hip for too long can cause a strain on back.
- Natural position for carrying baby is over the shoulder.

GENERAL POSTNATAL PHYSIOTHERAPY MANAGEMENT PROTOCOL

If woman had normal vaginal delivery, this protocol can be used. If she had any specific complication, treatment of that complication must be included in this protocol. Do not burden new mother with too many exercises.

1st Week

- Rest – as much as possible
- Iceing (15 – 20 minutes) and/or ultrasound for perineal pain
- Sit on the soft surface to prevent discomfort at the perineal region
- Gentle pelvic floor muscle exercises within limit of pain. (Quick contractions)
- TENS for after pains
- Gentle breast massage to prevent breast engorgement.
- Teach good posture for ADLs, during breastfeeding and while handling baby.
- Back care advice
- ATM
- Calf stretching
- Pelvic tilting exercises
- Cat and camel exercise.

2nd Week

- Pelvic floor muscle exercises (Quick contractions)
- Pelvic floor muscle relaxation - Opening up the hip rotators (Supine butterfly pose)

- Abdominal muscle strengthening (Check for the diastasis recti before starting abdominal strengthening)
- Head lift
- Leg sliding
- Iceing for perineal pain (15-20 minutes)
- Sit on the soft surface to prevent discomfort at the perineal region
- Rest
- Maintain good posture for ADLs, during breast feeding and while handling baby.
- Pelvic tilting exercises
- Cat and camel exercise
- Back care advice.

3rd Week

- Pelvic floor muscle exercises (Contract relax)
- Abdominal muscle strengthening
- Head lift
- Leg sliding
- Trunk curls
- Iceing for perineal pain (15 - 20 minutes)
- Rest
- Maintain good posture for ADLs, during breastfeeding and while handling baby.
- Pelvic tilting exercises
- Cat and camel exercise
- Back care advice.

4th Week

- Pelvic floor muscle exercises (Contract relax)
- Abdominal muscle strengthening
- Head lift
- Leg sliding
- Trunk curls
- Iceing for perineal pain (If needed) (15 - 20 minutes)
- Rest
- Maintain good posture for ADLs, during breast feeding and while handling baby.
- Pelvic tilting exercises
- Cat and camel exercise
- Back care advice.

5th Week

- Pelvic floor muscle strengthening exercises (contract relax – gradually increase the hold time)
- Abdominal muscle strengthening
- Head lift
- Leg sliding
- Trunk curls
- Diagonal curls
- Supine bicycle
- Maintain good posture for ADLs, during breastfeeding and while handling baby.
- Back care advice
- Pelvic tilting exercises
- Cat and camel
- Pelvic clock.

6th Week

- Pelvic floor muscle strengthening exercises (Elevator method)
- Abdominal muscle strengthening
- Head lift
- Leg sliding
- Trunk curls
- Diagonal curls
- Supine bicycle (Gradually progress by increasing the arc of cycling)
- Maintain good posture for ADLs, during breastfeeding and while handling baby
- Back care advice
- Pelvic tilting exercises
- Cat and camel
- Pelvic clock.

7th Week

- Pelvic floor muscle strengthening exercises (Elevator method)
- Abdominal muscle strengthening
- Head lift
- Leg sliding
- Trunk curls
- Diagonal curls
- Supine bicycle (Gradually progress by increasing the arc of cycling)

- Maintain good posture for ADLs, during breastfeeding and while handling baby.
- Back care advice
- Planks
- Pelvic tilting exercises
- Cat and camel
- Pelvic clock.

8th Week

- Pelvic floor muscle strengthening exercises (Elevator method – gradually increase the floors)
- Abdominal muscle strengthening
- Head lift
- Leg sliding
- Trunk curls
- Diagonal curls
- Supine bicycle (Gradually progress by increasing the arc of cycling)
- Maintain good posture for ADLs, during breast feeding and while handling baby.
- Back care advice
- Planks
- Pelvic tilting exercises
- Cat and camel
- Pelvic clock

STUDY QUESTIONS

1. What is diastasis recti? Explain about diagnosis and physiotherapy management of diastesis recti.
2. Tupler technique.
3. Importance of postnatal exercises.
4. Write in detail about physiotherapy management of musculoskeletal dysfunction during pregnancy.
5. Late postnatal complications and their physiotherapy management.
6. Identify the muscles of pelvic floor. Discuss the complications of weak pelvic floor muscle. Plan an exercise program to improve the same.
7. Care of back in postnatal period.
8. Draw the labeled diagram of abdominal muscles. Describe the various abdominal muscle exercises that are taught during antenatal and postnatal period.

9. Pelvic motion training.
10. Ergonomical advice in ADL of mother in postnatal period.
11. Justify the techniques and use of TENS in pregnancy, labor and postnatal period.

REFERENCES

1. Postpartum Fitness. The Permanent Medical Group Inc, 2009.
2. Advice for Physiotherapists and other Health Professionals. Association of Chartered Physiotherapists in Women's Health, Bathgate, 2016.
3. Lee W, Menard MD, Burns M. Guide to Fitness during and after Pregnancy in the CS. Ontario, 2003.
4. Postnatal Exercises, NHS Trust, Ashford and St. Peter's Hospitals, 2011.
5. Breastfeeding Positions and Postnatal Exercises for New Mothers. Bhailal Amin General Hospital, Baroda, 2008.
6. Physiotherapy after Child Birth. King Edward Memorials Hospital. Government of Western Australia. Women and Newborn Services, 2013.
7. Carolyn Kisner, Lynn Allen Colby. Therapeutic Exercise – Foundations and Techniques, 5th edition. Philadelphia, Margaret Biblis Publishers, 2007.
8. Lila Abbate, Secili DeStefano, Pamela Downey. Women's health across the lifespan, American Physical Therapy Association, Alexandria.
9. Margaret Polden, Jill Mantle, et al. Physiotherapy in Obstetrics and Gynecology, Elsevier Limited, 2004.
10. Exercise for Pregnancy, Childbirth and Postpartum, Department of Health North Dakota, 2009.
11. Physiotherapy before and after Childbirth. Women's and Children's Health Service, Department of Health, Government of Western Australia, 2006.
12. Pelvic Floor Exercises. The Royal Women's Hospital. Victoria Australia, 2010.
13. Ann Thompson et al. Tidy's Physiotherapy, 12th edition. Elsevier Publication, 31st March 1991.

CHAPTER 7

Physiotherapy after Cesarean Section

> **Chapter Outline**
> ➤ Indications of Cesarean Section
> ➤ Postoperative Physiotherapy Management
> ➤ Body Mechanics

INTRODUCTION

Cesarean section is also known as C-section is the use of surgery to deliver one or more babies. Usually it is performed when vaginal delivery might put the baby or mother at risk but sometimes it may be performed on request. According to studies, in those who are low risk the risk of death for cesarean section is 13 per 1,00,000 and for vaginal birth 3.5 per 1,00,000 in the developed world. After cesarean section woman needs some time for recovery. Exercises are the key to successful rehabilitation.[1]

Definition: It is a surgical procedure after the end of 28th weeks in which incisions are made through a woman's abdomen and uterus to deliver the fetus.[2,5]

The first surgery performed on a patient is referred as **"primary cesarean section"** and when the surgery is performed in subsequent pregnancies, it is called **"repeat cesarean section"**.[5]

INDICATIONS OF CESAREAN SECTION[2,5]

For indications of cesarean section see table 7.1

Table 7.1: Indications of cesarean section		
Fetal	Maternal-fetal	Maternal
Fetal distress (non-reassuring fetal heart pattern)	Obstructed labor	Previous cesarean delivery
Malposition and malpresentations	Placental abruption	Contracted/limited pelvic cavity or cephalopelvic disproportion

Contd...

Contd...

Fetal	Maternal-fetal	Maternal
Cord prolapsed–baby needs to be delivered immediately because prolapsed cord can cut off fetal oxygen supply.	Placenta previa (complete)	Pelvic mass causing obstruction
Macrosomia, congenital anomalies, multiple pregnancy	Perimortem	Active genital herpes virus
	Maternal-fetal disproportion	Elective cesarean section
	Failure to progress in labour	Abdominal cerclage
		Reconstructive vaginal surgery, e.g., fistula repair
		Vaginal obstruction (atresia, stenosis)
		Bad obstetric history–with recurrent fetal loss
		Medical gynecological disorders: Hypertensive disorders, uncontrolled diabetes, heart disease (coarctation of aorta, marfan's syndrome), mechanical obstruction (carcinoma cervix), following repair of vesicovaginal fistula, pulmonary condition, thrombocytopenia

POSTOPERATIVE PHYSIOTHERAPY MANAGEMENT

Day 1[2]

- Monitoring of vital signs and fundal status every 4-8 hours for 24 hours.
- Uterus massages and report extra lochia.
- Monitor fluids intake and output every four hours for 24 hours.
- Encourage early activity.
- Give fluids and soft diet after 6 hours.

Wound Support[4]

Coughing, sneezing or laughing may pull abdominal muscles. To make it more comfortable try to:
- Draw in abdominal muscles
- Support wound with pillow, towel or hands and apply gentle pressure.

If general anesthesia is used during a cesarean section, or if she do shallow breathing because of pain from the incision, secretions may pool in lungs. Women need to frequently take deep breaths, so that her lungs completely fill with air.[1]

Breathing Exercises[1,3,7]

- **Diaphragmatic breathing:** Support the incision with hands or a pillow then take a deep breathe.
- **Mid-chest expansion:** Place hands on lower ribs then take a deep breath and try to expand lungs under hands.
- **Upper chest expansion:** Place hands over upper chest then take a deep breath and try to expand lungs under hands.
- **Deep breathing:** Support the incision with hand or a pillow. Breathe in deeply and slowly through the nose. Ask her to fill lungs and imagine breathing deeply into abdomen. During breath in abdomen should move forward. Breathe out through mouth. During breathe out abdomen should move downwards. On the first day, do upto 5 breathes at a time.
- **Huffing and coughing exercises:** Do huffing, coughing and breathing exercises every hour until the woman can comfortably get in and out of bed and walk around.

Foot and Ankle Exercises[3,7]

These exercises will help to reduce or prevent pitting edema, varicose vain, cramp and improve circulation.

Knees must be relaxed for both exercises.
- Do alternate ankle plantar flexion and dorsiflexion movement.
- Circle both feet in each direction clockwise and anticlock wise.
- Repeat both of these exercises 30 seconds regularly.

Transcutaneous Electrical Nerve Stimulation (TENS)

TENS is used for pain relief usually after 8 hours. Studies show that use of TENS results in shorter hospital stay and less use of analgesic medications and therefore lesser complications of medications.

Electrode placement:
- 1 pair of electrode is placed on each side of T10 – L1.
- Another pair of electrode is placed at the side of incision.

Parameters:
- Frequency: 80-120 Hz
- Pulse duration: 150 µs
- Intensity: Minimal paresthesia

Duration: 1 hour 4 times/day.

Days 2 and 3

Repeat day one exercises and add:
Stand and walk tall with proper posture to prevent back pain.
Contract gluteal muscles during standing.

Moving around in Bed[4,7]

- Avoid twisting movements.
- To get out of bed, roll over onto side and let the legs drop over the edge of the bed. By using arms, push up in sitting position.
- To get into bed, sit as far as possible on the bed. Lower to the side using arms then gently lift legs up on the bed.
- In hospital, raise the head of the bed up to make above movements easier.

Posterior Pelvic Tilt[1,7]

In supine lying position with knees flexed and feet flat on the floor, flatten the lordotic curve against the bed and contract gluteal muscles. Hold this position for 3-5 seconds.

Leg Slides[1,3,6]

Patient position: Hook lying with posterior pelvic tilt.
Procedure: Hold the posterior pelvic tilt and slide one foot along the floor until the leg is straight or to the point at which she is unable to maintain the posterior pelvic tilt. Breathe in during this movement. Then slowly slide the leg back to the starting position and breathe out. Repeat same with the other leg.
  Repeat 5-10 times.

Hip Hike

In supine position, legs flat, and hike hip up and down. Repeat on both sides 5-10 times.[1]

Day 4 to 9

If woman can do above exercises without too much discomfort, begin the following exercises.

Pelvic Floor Muscle Exercises

For all women after the child birth including cesarean section, it is very important to exercise pelvic floor muscles.

Head Lift[1,6,7] (Fig. 7.1)

Patient position: Crook lying with hands crossed over midline.

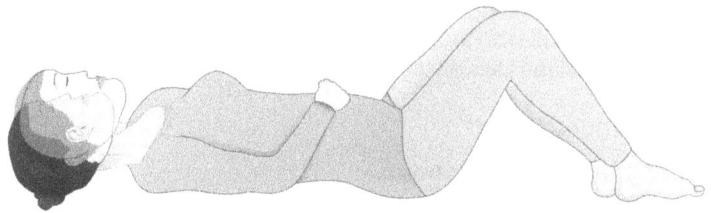

Figure 7.1: Head lift.

Procedure: Ask the woman to exhale and lift head off the floor. At the same time, her hands should support the incisions. Then ask the woman to lower her head slowly, inhale and relax.

Repeat 5 – 10 times.

Pelvic Rolling[1]

Patient position: Crook lying with shoulder abducted to 90 degrees.
Procedure: In crook-lying position, feet and shoulders flat on the supporting surface. Knees together then roll them from one side to the other. Feet should stay in the same place as knees roll from side to side.

Repeat 5 – 10 times.

Day 10

Do all of the exercises already listed and add:

Abdominal Exercises[7]

The most important function of abdominal muscles is to stabilize and protect spine and support the internal organs. These muscles get stretched and weak during pregnancy. Abdominal exercises will help to get these muscles back to their normal length and strength. Abdominal contractions are also helpful to maintain normal mobility of healing tissues and increase circulation to improve healing.

i. **Trunk curls**[1,6] **(Fig. 7.2)**
 Patient position: Crook lying with hands supporting incision site.

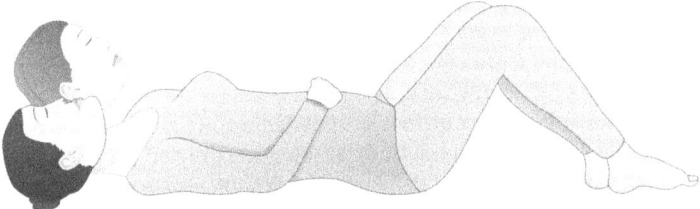

Figure 7.2: Trunk curls.

Procedure: Curl-downs and curl-ups are very good abdominal exercises. Ask woman to protect the incision with crossed hands while performing trunk curls. Lift head, chest, and shoulders slightly off the bed (until the inferior angle of scapula clears the bed surface). Repeat this exercise 10 times. Breathe out while lifting head up.

ii. **Diagonal curls**[1,6]
 Patient position: Crook lying with hands supporting incision site.
 Procedure: Diagonals are helpful to strengthen oblique muscles. Lift one shoulder towards the opposite knee as she curls up and down and protects the incision site with crossed hands. Repeat 10 times.
 Caution: If woman is having diastasis recti, give more support to the area while exercising. While doing both of the above exercises, lift only head off the floor and then cross hands over abdomen.[1] (For more details check "Diastasis recti" Chapter no. 6)

BODY MECHANICS[1,3]

After a Cesarean, women may lean forward to protect her incision. Ask her to support the incision and start walking within the first 12–18 hours. It will help to improve digestion and decrease muscle stiffness. Walking and gentle exercise will not pull apart the incision but exercise and activity will help healing by increasing circulation.

- **Avoid sitting on soft chairs:** Soft chairs require more effort while getting up from the chair and usually do not give proper back support. Advice woman to sit in a firm, straight back chair and not to slouch or arch lower back. Put the pillow or cushion near the lower back and hips for the extra support.
- **To get up from the bed:** Do not get up by bending at the waist. Slowly roll to one side and swing legs over the edge of the bed, one at a time. Try to push up upper body with the elbow on the side she is on and then get up.

- **Go up and down stairs slowly:** Take one step at a time so that she will not get tired. Use thigh and hip muscles while stair climbing and descending. Keep back straight and weight over feet.
- **When bending over:** Keep one foot in front of the other. Flex knees and lower the trunk. Keep lower back slightly curved. Legs should take most of the body weight.
- **To lift an object:** Put one foot in front of the other and keep the object as close as possible to the body or touching the body at about waist height. Lift small weight to avoid overexertion.
- **Reach for high objects:** Avoid overstretching and use the stool to reach any high object. Keep frequently used objects at closer reach.

STUDY QUESTIONS

1. Explain about the proper body mechanics after the cesarean section.
2. Postnatal exercises following cesarean section.
3. 30-year-old female had a cesarean section for the delivery of twins 4 days ago. The babies weighed 3 kilos and she reports "gapping" between her stomach muscles. Assess her abdominal muscle and give her appropriate advice and exercise to return normal support mechanics for the pelvis and lumbar spine.

REFERENCES

1. Ceren Gursen et al. Effects of exercise and kinesio tapeing on abdominal recovery in women with cesarean section: a pilot randomized controlled trial. Metarnal - Fetal medicine, 2015.
2. Rulisa Stephen et al. Clinical Treatment Guidelines: Gynecology and Obstetrics. Ministry of Health, 2012.
3. After your Cesarean Birth: What you can do, BC Women's Hospital and Health Centre, 2009.
4. Your recovery after childbirth. NHS trust–Oxford University Hospitals, 2016.
5. Dutta DC, Konar H. DC Dutta's Textbook of Obstetrics. Jaypee Brothers Medical Publishers, 8th edition, 2015.
6. Kisner C, Colby LA. Therapeutic Exercise – Foundations and Techniques, 5th edition. Philadelphia, Margaret Biblis Publishers, 2007.
7. Ann Thompson et al. Tidy's Physiotherapy, 12th edition. Elsevier Publication, 1991.

CHAPTER 8

Painless Labor

> **Chapter Outline**
> ➤ Epidural Anesthesia

INTRODUCTION

Labor is hard work. Labor is an end to pregnancy and a beginning for a new human life in the family.

One of the most severe pains that a woman experiences in her lifetime is labor pain. Almost every woman bears the labor pain. If women will get chance, every woman wants to get rid of the labor pain as soon as possible. There are many myths and controversies about the relief of labor pain. The concept of modern labor analgesia was born in the early nineteenth century. The concept of regional anesthesia came during mid twentieth century. The most suitable method of anesthesia during labor is epidural. In this method, the anesthetist injects pain relieving medication through a small tube in the back.[1,2]

EPIDURAL ANESTHESIA

Epidural anesthesia is an advance in pain management during labor. With the help of epidural anesthesia, a pregnant woman has a comfortable labor. It is a regional anesthesia in which low doses of local anesthetic are administered near the spinal cord in the spinal canal to provide a continues T10–L1 sensory block during the labor.[2]

Areas Affected

It gives anesthetic effect below the waist level, but the movements are not impaired.

Time of Anesthesia

It is administered in active labor. It can be given as a single injection or in multiple doses through epidural catheter by an anesthetist.

Advantages

- Safe and effective.
- It gives almost complete relief from pain and also allows the woman to be mobile.
- No postpartum headache. (In case of spinal anesthesia, woman will have postpartum headache).
- Woman is conscious and alert during the labor.
- An instrumental delivery can also perform under this anesthesia, if needed.
- If there is need for cesarean section, the anesthetic effect can be refilled through the epidural catheter.

Disadvantages

- It can cause sudden drop in the blood pressure.
- Because of pelvic floor relaxation, baby's head may not rotate and forceps application may be required.
- Slight increased chances of instrumental and cesarean deliveries.

Fluid Preloading

Fluid preloading is beneficial before introducing labor epidurals when fetus is at increased risk. Routine use of fluid preloading may lead to prolonged labor due to decreased uterine activity.

STUDY QUESTIONS

1. Explain in detail about epidural anesthesia and its importance.
2. Side effects and complications of epidural anesthesia.

REFERENCES

1. Bajwa SK, Bajwa SJ, Singh K et al. Painless labor: how far have we travelled?, Sri Lanka Journal of Obstetrics and Gynecology. 2010;32(4): 93-98.
2. Dehghanpisheh L, Sabetian G, Fatahi Z. Painless delivery: Knowledge and attitude of obstetricians and midwives, The Professional Medical Journal. 2016:67-71.

CHAPTER 9

Common Medical Problems in Pregnancy

Chapter Outline
- Iron Deficiency Anemia
- Pregnancy-induced Hypertension or Pre-eclampsia
- Eclampsia
- Polyhydramnios
- Premature Rupture of Membrane
- Intrauterine Fetal Death
- Gestational Diabetes Mellitus

INTRODUCTION

During pregnancy many women suffer from medical problems and complications. As a physiotherapist if we find any of these problems or complications, we have to recognize that and immediately refer the patient to concern doctor for appropriate treatment. We work in a multidisciplinary team so referring the patient is also most important part of treatment and safety of patient.

IRON DEFICIENCY ANEMIA[1,2]

Anemia is defined as a hemoglobin level below 11 g/dL during the first and third trimester and below 10.5 g/dL during the second trimester. If woman is having pre-existing anemia, it can aggravate during pregnancy. Anemia increases the risk of premature birth and intrauterine growth retardation.

Symptoms
- Pallor of conjunctiva, mucous membrane, palms and sole of feet
- Fatigue

- Dizziness
- Tachycardia
- Heart murmur
- Signs of serious illness: Intense pallor, tiredness, difficulty in breathing, hemoglobin levels below 7 g/dL.

PREGNANCY-INDUCED HYPERTENSION OR PRE-ECLAMPSIA[1-3]

During pregnancy blood pressure will change than non-pregnant levels. Normally blood pressure (BP) slightly decreases during pregnancy. The hormone relaxin will relax the wall of blood vessels. This will reduce blood pressure in first and second trimester. During pregnancy blood pressure 140/90 mm Hg or above is considered as high blood pressure. To conform hypertension check BP several times and at resting position. Chronic hypertension is defined as high blood pressure before pregnancy or before 20 weeks of last menstrual period.

Pregnancy-induced hypertension (PIH) with proteinuria is known as pre-eclampsia. It can increase the risk of fetal growth retardation, fetal distress, fetal death, placental abruption and eclampsia. High blood pressure is most visible sign of pre-eclampsia but it is a complex disease affecting multiple organs including liver and kidney. The goal of antihypertensive treatment is to prevent maternal complications. Treatment is administered if systolic BP is ≥160 mm Hg or diastolic BP is ≥ 110 mm Hg. During every visit it is very important to measure maternal BP and the objective is to maintain blood pressure about 140/90 mm Hg. Antihypertensive treatment should be administered with precaution. It is important to preserve placental perfusion and avoid excessive fall in maternal BP.

Symptoms

- BP ≥ 140/90 mm Hg and proteinuria (1+ or more on dipstick test)
- Dark urine, low urine output, edema of hands or legs that appears suddenly or worsen rapidly.
- In woman with proteinuria without hypertension consider urinary tract infection or renal disease. In this type of cases monitor continuously to detect pre-eclampsia in early stage.

Common Medical Problems in Pregnancy

PIH can be classified as given in table 9.1.

Table 9.1:	Classification of PIH
Mild	A BP upto 140/90 mm Hg without proteinuria.
Moderate	A BP upto 160/110 mm Hg without proteinuria. In absence of proteinuria, PIH is rarely dangerous to mother and fetus.
Severe	A BP more than 160/110 mm Hg and presence of proteinuria.

Severe Pre-eclampsia

- Systolic BP is ≥160 mm Hg or diastolic BP is ≥ 110 mm Hg, remains elevated in spite of antihypertensive treatment.
- Proteinuria (3+ or more on dipstick test or more than 5 g/day).
- Oliguria (Urine output < 400 mL/day or < 30 mL/hour).
- Hyperreflaxia (overactive knee jerk, spasm or twitching)
- Nausea, vomiting, epigastric pain
- Facial and pulmonary edema
- Severe headache and it is not relieved by medicine.
- Buzzing in ear
- Visual disturbances.

The HELLP syndrome (hemolysis, elevated liver enzyme, low platelets) is a potential life threatening complication for mother and fetus both.

ECLAMPSIA

Convulsion occurs during third trimester of pregnancy mainly followed by pre-eclampsia. Eclampsia can also occur within 48 hours after delivery. Consider other causes of convulsion like cerebral malaria and meningitis as their incidence is increased in pregnant woman.[1,2]

POLYHYDRAMNIOS[1]

Excess amniotic fluid, more than two liters at term is considered as polyhydramnios. It can be due to fetal anomalies.

Symptoms

Acute Polyhydramnios

Mainly associated with fetal malformation or complicated twin pregnancy.
- In second trimester of pregnancy
- Rapid increase in size of uterus

- Painful abdomen, dyspnea
- Distended hard uterus
- Fetus cannot be palpated.

Do not intervene in this situation, let the patient abort or deliver spontaneously.

Chronic Polyhydramnios

- In third trimester of pregnancy
- More moderate increase in size of uterus
- Fetus cannot be palpated
- Receding head on vaginal examination, fluid wave
- Fetal heart beat muffled.

PREMATURE RUPTURE OF MEMBRANE[1,5]

Discharge of amniotic fluid before the onset of labor. It can be due to rupture or leak of amniotic sac. There is risk of preterm birth if rupture occurs before 37 weeks of last menstrual period.

Differential diagnosis: Urinary incontinence, leukorrhea, expulsion of mucus plug.

INTRAUTERINE FETAL DEATH[1,5]

Fetal death occurs before the onset of labor.

Symptoms

- Absent or cessation of fetal movements
- Fundal height small for gestation age, fundal height decrease than prior visit
- Absence of fetal heart sound
- Breast engorgement which indicates termination of pregnancy.

After delivery mothers are at risk of psychological problems like postpartum depression after stillbirth. Psychological support is must in hospital and post partum period.

GESTATIONAL DIABETES MELLITUS (GDM)

Diabetes is the most common medical complication of pregnancy. It can be classified as, those who have diabetes before pregnancy, "Pregestational" and those who diagnosed after pregnancy, "gestational".

GDM is defined as, the carbohydrate intolerance of variable severity with onset or first recognized during pregnancy. It usually presents after the beginning of second trimester and resolves after birth, but woman have significantly increased risk of developing diabetes mellitus type II particularly in the first 5 years postpartum.

During pregnancy the placenta releases hormones which aid the baby's growth. These hormones block the action of the mother's insulin, creating insulin resistance. Due to insulin resistance the mother must release 2-3 times more insulin than usual. If the mother cannot release the required amount of insulin, gestational diabetes develops. During gestational diabetes the mother's high blood glucose levels cross the placenta and create high blood glucose levels in the baby. The baby responds by releasing extra insulin from their pancreas. This leads to a bigger and fatter baby, which can lead to the premature delivery of baby and increases the risk of pre-eclampsia and cesarean delivery. It also stresses the baby's immature pancreas and increases the risk of the baby developing type II diabetes later in life.

High Risk Patients[4,6]

- Previous pregnancy with gestational diabetes
- Overweight or obese
- Excessive weight gain during pregnancy
- Family history of diabetes
- High weight babies born from a previous pregnancy
- A history of stillbirth or infants with congenital abnormalities
- Maternal age more than 30 years
- A history of repeated or persistent urinary tract infection
- Poor obstetric history including hypertension, eclampsia, hydramnios, etc.
- Short stature
- Smoking.

Risk to Fetus[4,5,6]

- Macrosomia: It is a condition in which baby grows too large due to excess insulin crossing the placenta. A large baby can make vaginal delivery difficult and increase the risk of injury to the baby during birth process.
- Hypoglycemia: Hypoglycemia or low blood sugar can develop shortly after birth due to high insulin levels. Controlling maternal blood sugar levels help to lower the risk of hypoglycemia to fetus.
- Jaundice
- High neonatal body fat percentage

Fetal problems associated with maternal hyperglycemia according to trimesters of gestation are given in Table 9.2.

Table 9.2: Fetal problems associated with maternal hyperglycemia according to trimesters of gestation

First trimester	Second trimester	Third trimester
Malformations	Hypertrophic cardiomyopathy	Hypoglycemia
Growth retardation	Polyhydramnios	Hypocalcemia
Fetal wastage	Erythremia	Hyperbilirubinemia
	Placental insufficiency	Respiratory distress syndrome
	Pre-eclampsia	Macrosomia
	Fetal loss	Hypomagnesemia
	Low IQ	Intrauterine death

Diagnosis

GDM can only be confirmed by an abnormal glucose tolerance test. According to world health organization:
- A fasting blood glucose level >7 mmol/L
- A blood glucose level 2 hours after 75 g glucose drink >7.8 mmol/L.

PHYSIOTHERAPY MANAGEMENT[4,5]

Maintaining healthy weight is very important in prevention and management of GDM. Modify diet and lifestyle can help to control weight and also the blood glucose levels. Exercise makes the cells in body more receptive to insulin, resulting in improved insulin sensitivity for 48 hours after exercise. Advice to do exercise on most days of the week with no more than 48 hours between exercise sessions as the effects of exercise on insulin sensitivity only last 48 hours after exercise. If the gestational diabetes is controlled, the risks to both baby and mother are reduced. The lifestyle changes made during pregnancy should be continued even after the birth. This will help to reduce the risk of type II diabetes and obesity later in life.

If woman had following symptoms during exercises, exercises must be discontinued:
- Vaginal bleeding
- Dizziness
- Dyspnea
- Headache
- Chest pain

Common Medical Problems in Pregnancy

- Muscle weakness
- Calf pain or swelling
- Decreased fetal movements
- Amniotic fluid leakage

Following exercises have shown to stabilize or lower the glucose levels. These exercises must be done for 30 – 60 minutes, at least 3 times per week. The gap between exercises must not be more than 48 hours.

- Brisk walking
- Recumbent bicycling
- Arm ergometer
- Moderate intensity resistance exercise
- Moderate intensity aerobics for 20 – 30 minutes
- Swimming
- During postnatal period, mothers are advised to breastfeed her baby. Breastfeeding is also helpful to lower the fasting blood glucose level in mothers.
- Yoga, pranayama
- Pilates.

Physiotherapy Management for the Prevention of GDM

According to studies, regular light to moderate exercise, for 30–40 minutes 3 times per week during pregnancy can prevent the GDM.

Safe exercises during pregnancy to prevent GDM are:

- Static cycling: According to studies 30 minutes of cycling 3 times per day in early pregnancy decreases the chances of getting GDM even in overweight or obese woman.
- Walking
- Low impact aerobics
- Modified yoga and pilates
- Strength training.

STUDY QUESTIONS

1. Classify pregnancy-induced hypertension and explain in detail about pre-eclampsia.
2. Gestational diabetes.
3. 19-year-old primigravida comes in emergency at 32 weeks of gestation. She is complaining of blurring of vision and gross edema. On examination her blood pressure is 170 / 115 mm Hg. What is the most likely diagnosis?

a. Hypertension
b. Renal disease
c. Eclampsia
d. Pre-eclampsia.

REFERENCES

1. Coutin AS. Essential Obstetrics and Newborn care, 2015 edition.
2. Beckmann Charles RB, Ling FW, Barzansky BM. Obstetrics and Gynecology, 6th edition. The American College of Obstetricians and Gynecologists, New York, 2010.
3. Diana Hamilton–Fairley. Obstetrics and Gynecology, 2nd edition, Blackwell Publications, 2004.
4. Krishna Murthy E, Pavlić-Renar I, Metelko Z. Diabetes and Pregnancy, Vuk Vrhovac Institute, University Clinic for Diabetes. 2002:131-46.
5. Kisner C, Colby LA. Therapeutic Exercise–Foundations and Techniques, 5th edition. Philadelphia, Margaret Biblis Publishers. 2007.
6. Dutta DC, Konar H. DC Dutta's Textbook of Obstetrics, 8th edition. Jaypee Brothers Medical Publishers, 2015.

10

Water Birth

Chapter Outline
- Benefits of Water Birth
- Risks of Water Birth
- Contraindications for Water Birth

INTRODUCTION

Giving birth in a tub of warm water (around 37 degree Celsius) is known as water birth. Some women choose to have labor in the water and some decide to stay in the water for the delivery also. The baby was in the amniotic fluid for nine months so birthing baby in a similar environment is less stressful for both the mother and baby. Water birth must occur under the supervision of a qualified obstetrician.

BENEFITS OF WATER BIRTH

Benefits for Woman

- Warm water is soothing and help woman to be relax and comfortable during labor and delivery.
- Water increases the energy of woman.
- Buoyancy reduces woman's body weight and allows her to move freely and also helps to adopt new comfortable positioning during labor.
- Buoyancy promotes more effective uterine contractions and helps to improve blood circulation. It will result in better oxygenation of the uterine muscles, less painful labor for the woman and more oxygen for the baby.

- There are chances of increase in blood pressure during labor and delivery due to anxiety. Immersion in warm water as in water birth will help to reduce or maintain blood pressure.
- The water helps to reduce stress-related hormones and allows the woman to produce natural pain killer like endorphins.
- Water makes perineum more elastic and relaxed so it reduces the incidence and severity of perineum tear and the need for an episiotomy.
- If woman is physically and mentally relaxed during labor and delivery, she will be able to focus on the birthing process.

Benefits for Baby

- Water birth provides same environment as the amniotic sac.
- It reduces the birth stress and increases comfort level in baby.

RISKS OF WATER BIRTH

According to some studies, mortality rate is same in water birth and conventional birth. During water birth, when water enters into the woman's blood stream, water embolism can occur. The British Medical Journal is 95% confident in the safety of mother and baby during water birth but there is risk of water aspiration. If the baby experience stress in the birth canal or if the umbilical cord is kinked or twisted, the baby might gasp air with the inhaling water. This is very rare because normally babies do not inhale until they are exposed to air. Baby will continue to receive oxygen through the umbilical cord until they start to breathe on their own or until the umbilical cord is cut. The risk is that the umbilical cord can break while the baby is brought to the surface of the water. To prevent this, have precaution while lifting the baby up to the surface of water.

CONTRAINDICATIONS FOR WATER BIRTH

- Herpes
- Excessive bleeding or maternal infection
- Preterm labor
- Toxemia or pre-eclampsia

Glossary

- **Atresia**: Absence or abnormal narrowing of an opening or passage in the body.
- **Ballottement**: Diagnostic technique using palpation: A floating fetus when tapped or pushed, moves away and then returns to touch the examiner's hand.
- **Bratox-Hicks contraction/sign**: Intermittent weak contractions of uterus occurring during middle of pregnancy in first pregnancy and earlier in subsequent pregnancies. It is also known as false labor pains.
- **Bruising**: Injury of underlying soft tissue or bone without breaking the skin.
- **Chadwick sign**: Bluish discoloration of vagina, cervix and labia that is visible from approximately the fourth weeks of pregnancy, caused by increased vascularity.
- **Chloasma**: Increased pigmentation over bridge of nose and cheeks of pregnant woman and some women taking contraceptives. Also known as "Mask of Pregnancy".
- **Colostrum**: It is the first milk produced during pregnancy. It is the fluid in the acini cells of the breasts present from early pregnancy to the early postnatal period; rich in antibodies, which provide protection to the breastfed newborn from many diseases; high in protein and laxative acting, which speeds the elimination of meconium and helps loosen mucus.
- **Conjunctiva**: The mucous membrane that covers the front of eye and lines of eyelids.
- **Convulsion**: Sudden, violent and irregular movement of body due to involuntary muscle contraction.
- **Choriocarcinoma**: A malignant, tropoblastic tumor of the uterus which originates in the fetal chorion. The abnormal cells start in the tissue that would normally become the placenta.
- **Cyanosis**: An abnormal bluish discoloration of the skin and mucous membrane due to poor circulation or inadequate oxygen supply.

- **Dependent edema**: Edema of the lower part of the body relative to the heart. It is affected by gravity and position. Lower limbs are affected if person is standing and buttocks are affected if individual is in supine position.
- **Dieresis**: Increased or excessive production of urine.
- **Dysmenorrhea**: Painful Menstruation.
- **Dyspnea**: Labored or difficult breathing.
- **Eclampsia**: A condition characterized by convulsion or coma in a pregnant woman suffering from hypertension or pre-eclampsia.
- **Ectopic pregnancy**: It is one of the complication of pregnancy in which embryo attaches outside the uterus.
- **Edema**: Swelling caused by abnormal excess fluid in body tissue.
- **Episiotomy**: Surgical incision of the perineum and the posterior vaginal wall during second stage of labor to quickly enlarge the opening for the baby to pass through.
- **Epulis**: Tumorlike benign lesion of the gums seen in pregnant woman.
- **Erythroblastosis fetalis**: It is hemolytic anemia in the fetus and new-born caused by Rh incompatibility between maternal and fetal blood. Typically occurs when Rh negative mother inherits Rh positive blood from the father.
- **Funic souffle**: Soft blowing sound produced by blood rushing through the umbilical vessels and synchronous with the fetal heart sounds.
- **Gestation**: The process or period of developing inside the womb between conception and birth.
- **Gestational diabetes**: Woman without diabetes develops high blood sugar levels during pregnancy.
- **Glucosuria**: Excretion of glucose into the urine.
- **Goodell sign**: Softening of cervix, a probable sign of pregnancy, occurring as early as 6th week.
- **Gravida**: A woman who is pregnant.
- **Hemolysis**: Abnormal destruction or rupture (lysis) of red blood cells either intra or extravascular.
- **Hemorrhoids**: Swollen veins at the lowest part of rectum and anus.
- **Hegar sign**: Softening of lower uterine segment may be present at second and third month of pregnancy. It is palpated during bimanual examination.
- **Human chorionic gonadotropin (hCG)**: Hormone which is produced by chorionic villi, the biologic maker in pregnancy tests.
- **Labor**: Series of events that take place in the genital organs in an effort to expel the fetus, placenta and membranes out of the womb through the vagina into the outer world is called labor.

Glossary

- **Lochia**: It is the vaginal discharge for the first fortnight during puerperium.
- **Leukorrhea**: White or yellowish mucus discharge from the cervical canal or the vagina that may be normal physiological or caused by pathologic states of vagina and endocervix.
- **Lightening**: It is the sensation of decreased abdominal distention produced by uterine descent into the pelvic cavity as the fetal presenting part settles into the pelvis; usually occurs 2 weeks before the onset of labor in nulliparas woman.
- **Linea nigra**: It is the line of darker pigmentation seen in some women during the later part of pregnancy that appears on the middle of the abdomen and extends from the symphysis pubis towards the umbilicus.
- **Marfan's syndrome**: It is the genetic disorder that affects connective tissue and cause problem in eyes, joint and heart.
- **Macrosomic neonate**: Excessive intrauterine growth. A new born with excessive birth weight. According to American College of Obstetrics and Gynecology and the World Health Organization, newborns weighing more than 4000 g are considered to be macrosomic.
- **Menarche**: First menstrual cycle in female humans.
- **Menstruation**: Regular discharge of the blood and mucosal tissue from the inner lining of the non pregnant uterus through the vagina.
- **Molar pregnancy/Hydatidiform mole**: It is a rare abnormal form of pregnancy in which non-viable fertilized egg implants in the uterus and will fail to come to term.
- **Montgomery tubercles**: It is the small, nodular prominences (sebaceous glands) on the areolas around the nipples of the breasts that enlarge during pregnancy and lactation.
- **Multigravida**: The woman who has previously been pregnant. She may have aborted or have delivered a visible baby.
- **Multipara**: The woman who has completed two or more pregnancies to the stage of viability or more.
- **Muscle twitching**: Abnormal uncontrolled muscle contraction of muscle group that is supplied by a single motor nerve fiber.
- **Neonate**: A newborn child.
- **Nulligravida**: The woman who is not now and never has been pregnant.
- **Nullipara**: The woman who has never completed a pregnancy to the stage of viability. She may or may not have aborted previously.
- **Oliguria**: Production of abnormally small amount of urine (less than 400 mL/day).
- **Parturient**: The woman in labor.

- **Perimortem**: At or near the time of death.
- **Placenta praevia**: It is the obstetric complication in which placenta covers partial or whole opening in the mother's cervix.
- **Pollakiuria**: Frequent abnormal urination during day.
- **Polycystic ovary syndrome**: It is a hormonal disorder causing enlarged ovaries with small cysts on the outer edges.
- **Polyuria**: Production of abnormally large volume of diluted urine which is equal or more than 2.5 liters per day secondary to an abnormality of urine concentration.
- **Post-coital**: Occurring or done after the sexual intercourse.
- **Pre-eclampsia**: It is a condition characterized by high blood pressure in pregnant woman who has not experienced high blood pressure before.
- **Primigravida**: The woman who is pregnant for the first time.
- **Primipara**: The woman who has delivered one visible child. (Even if there are more than one child like, twins or triplets)
- **Proteinuria**: Presence of excess protein in urine (more than 5 g/day)
- **Puerpera**: The woman who has just given birth.
- **Puerperium**: The time immediately after the birth of the baby.
- **Quickening**: The first moment in pregnancy when the pregnant woman starts to feel movements of the fetus in uterus usually occurs between weeks 16 and 20 of gestation.
- **Sacral promontory**: The inwardly projecting anterior part of the body of the first sacral vertebra.
- **Striae gravidarum**: It is "Stretch marks" shining reddish lines caused by stretching of the skin, often found on the abdomen, thighs, and breasts during pregnancy.
- **Ureter**: The duct by which urine passes from kidney to bladder.
- **Uterine contraction**: Rhythmic tightening and shortening of uterine muscles.
- **Uterine souffle**: Soft, blowing sound made by the blood in the arteries of the pregnant uterus and synchronous with the maternal pulse.

Index

Page numbers followed by *f* refer to figure, and *t* refer to table

A

Abdomen, painful 120
Adenohypophysis 9
Allergic reaction 34
Amenorrhea 28, 30
Amniotic fluid 12, 47, 125
    discharge of 120
    leakage 123
Anatomical changes during
        pregnancy 11, 18*t*
Anemia 117
    history of 33
    iron deficiency 117
Anesthesia
    epidural 115
    regional 115
    time of 116
Ankle
    dorsiflexion 97
    edema 35
Anticoagulant therapy 97
Anulom vilom 54
Arms 51
    ergometer 123
Arthritis 65
Asanas 61, 62
Asthma 33, 39
Atresia 127
Autism spectrum disorders 31
Autonomic nervous system, pelvic
        part of 7

B

Back and pelvis
    care 55
    pain 55
Back labor, positions for 78
Back pain
    during pregnancy 55
    postural 93, 100
Backward stretch 52, 52*f*
    with fitness ball 52, 52*f*
Ballottement 30, 127

Bicycle in supine 99
Bladder irritability 28
Bleeding
    excessive 126
    vaginal 46, 122
Blood 12, 47
    gases 15
    loss in delivery 12
    pressure 14, 46, 118
        diastolic 18
        systolic 14, 18, 119
    tests 29
    transfusion 34
    volume 12, 13, 85
Body mass index 37
Body mechanics 113
Bony pelvis, female 1
Bowel movements 85
Bratox-Hicks contraction 30, 36, 127
Breasts 12, 47
    changes 29, 30, 85
    discomfort 28
    engorgement 97
    examination 35
Breath hold 50
Breathing 72
    diaphragmatic 110
    during labor 73*t*
    exercises 49, 110
Brisk walking 123
Bruising 127
Bulbocavernosus 17
Buttocks, contraction of 50

C

Calf
    pain 97, 123
    stretching 53
    swelling 123
Capillary refill time 35
Cardiac output 18, 66
Cardiomyopathy, hypertrophic 122
Cardiovascular physiology 18

Cardiovascular system 13
Carpal tunnel syndrome 99
Cat and camel exercise 51
Cervical
    dilation phase 70
    lordosis 25
    polyps 30
Cesarean section 108
    indications of 108, 108t
    physiotherapy after 108
    primary 108
    repeat 108
Chadwick's sign 28, 30, 127
Childhood disease 33
Chloasma 29, 127
Choriocarcinoma 127
Chronic disease 33
Coccydynia 94
Coccygeal plexus 6
Coccygeus 19
Colostrum 127
Compressor urethrae 19
Congenital diseases 33
Conjunctiva 127
    pallor of 117
Convulsion 127
Corpus luteum 9
Corticosteroid binding globulin 16
Coughing exercises 110
Creatinine clearance 19
Crushed ice 89
Cryotherapy 89
C-section 108
Curve of Carus 3
Cyanosis 127

D

Dance with belly lift 77f
Dandasana 54
Deep breathing 110
    exercise 50
Deep urogenital diaphragm layer 19
Deep vein thrombosis 97
Delivery 85
    vaginal 12, 108
Diabetes 33, 39, 120
    mellitus, gestational 120, 128

Diagonal curls 113
Diarrhea 46
Diastasis recti 90, 90f, 93t
    corrective exercises for 92
    mild 92
    minor 92
    muscle assessment 40
    presence of 91
    severe 92
Dieresis 128
Dizziness 118, 122
Doppler ultrasound 30
Dysmenorrhea 32, 128
Dyspnea 120, 122, 128

E

Ear, buzzing in 119
Eclampsia 119, 128
Edema 47, 96, 128
    facial 119
    pulmonary 119
Egg cells 8
Electrode placement 74, 111
Endocrine
    problems 30
    system 15
Epilepsy 33
Episiotomy 128
Epulis 128
Erythremia 122
Erythroblastosis fetalis 128
Erythrocyte sedimentation rate 18
Estrogen 9, 10
Exercise
    abdominal 56, 112
    during pregnancy 44, 44t
    benefits of 45
    guidelines for 43
    elevator 101
    foot and ankle 57, 110
    postural 87
Expected date of delivery 32
    calculation of 37
Expiratory reserve volume 19
Expulsion 71
Extension 71

Index

F

Fallopian tube 11
False pelvis 2, 2f
Fatigue 28, 30, 117
Feet 51
Female breast during pregnancy, changes in 8f
Fetal death 120
Fetal descent positions 71, 71f
Fetal loss 122
Fetal movements 47, 123
    loss of 46
    palpated 30
    visible 30
Fetal problems 122
Fetal stethoscope 30
Fetal wastage 122
Fetus 12, 47, 120
    metabolic needs of 12
    visualization of 30
Fever 46
Fitness exercises, recommendations for 63
Flexion 71
Fluid 12, 47
    preloading 116
Follicle stimulating hormone 9
Follicular phase 10
Food poisoning 30
Functional residual capacity 18
Fundal grip 36, 37f
Fundal height 47
Funic souffle 128

G

Gait 25
    parameters observed during pregnancy 26t
    types of 26
Gas 30
Gastric
    acid secretion 19
    emptying 19
Gastrointestinal system 15
Gastrointestinal virus 30
General postnatal physiotherapy management protocol 103
Genital organs 69
Gestation 128
    trimesters of 122
Gestational age 30, 47
Getting off and on bed 60, 60f
Glands
    adrenal 16
    endometrial 10
Glomerular filtration rate 15, 19
Glucose metabolism 15
Glucosuria 128
Glycosuria 19
Goodell's sign 28, 30, 128
Graafian follicle 9
Gravida 128
Gravity, center of 22
Greater pelvis 2
Growth retardation 122
Gynecological procedures 34

H

Head and neck 51
Head lift 112, 112f, 92, 92f, 93, 93f
Headache 46, 122
    severe 119
Heart 13
    disease 33
    murmur 118
    rate 14, 18, 48, 66, 85
        fetal 29, 30, 36, 48
        range 48t
    sounds, fetal 30
    tones, fetal 30
Heartburn 19
Hegar's sign 28, 30, 128
Hematocrit 13
Hematological parameters 18
Hematology 12
Hematoma, vaginal 88
Hemolysis 128
    elevated liver enzyme, low platelets syndrome 119
Hemorrhoids 128
Hepatitis 33
    A infection 33
    acute viral 33
    B 33
    C 33
    E infection 33

Hereditary diseases 33
Herniation 91
Herpes 126
Hip
   extensors 40
   flexors 39
   gluteals 40
   hike 111
   mobility 100
Homan's sign 97
Hormonal changes 85
Hormone 9, 64
   adrenocorticotropic 16
Hot water bath 98
Huffing exercises 110
Human chorionic gonadotropin 128
Human milk 7
Hydatidiform mole 129
Hydrotherapy 61
Hyperbilirubinemia 122
Hyperglycemia, maternal 122
Hyperreflexia 119
Hypertension 39, 118
   pregnancy-induced 118, 119t
Hypocalcemia 122
Hypoglycemia 121, 122
Hypomagnesemia 122

I

Ice cube massage 89
Iliococcygeus 19
Immunological tests 29
Infection, maternal 33, 126
Inspiratory reserve volume 18
Internal iliac arteries supplies,
      branches of anterior division
      of 5
Intrauterine
  death 122
  fetal death 120
  growth
     restriction 46
     retardation 47, 117
Ischiocavernosus 17
Ischiococcygeus 19

J

Jacquemier's sign 28
Jaundice 121
Joints
   laxity 24
   tightening of 85

K

Katichakrasana 54, 61
Kick charts 47
Knee
   chest 80f
   extension 97
   hyperextension 25
Kneeling 79, 79f, 87
   chair supported 80f

L

Labor 69-72, 85, 115, 128
   first stage of 75
   initiation of 69
   painless 115
   physiotherapy during 69
   positions in 75
   second stage of 80
   stages of 69
Last normal menstrual period 32
Lateral grip 36, 37f
Laura Mitchell method 54
Legs 51
   slides 99, 111
Leopold maneuver 36, 37f
Lesser pelvis 2
Leukemia, childhood acute
      lymphoblastic 31
Leukorrhea 120, 129
Levator ani 20
Levator scapulae 39
Lie of baby 47
Lifting posture 58, 58f
Linea alba 90
Linea nigra 17, 129
Lochia 129
Low impact aerobic exercises 49, 123
Low intensity 88

Index

Lower back
　deep muscles of 39
　irregular contractions in 78
　pain 78
　　symptoms of 94
　stretches 55, 52*f*
Lower esophageal sphincter pressure 19
　minus gastric pressure 15
Lumbar lordosis 25
Lumbar spine 23
　during pregnancy, biomechanics of 23
　lordosis of 24*f*
Lunge 78*f*
Luteal phase 11
Luteinizing hormone 9, 10

M

Macrosomia 121, 122
Macrosomic neonate 129
Magnetic resonance imaging 29
Malformations 122
Malnutrition 30
Mammary glands 7
　during pregnancy, changes in 7
Marfan's syndrome 129
Mass, abdominal 24*f*
Massage 54, 61
　perineal 61
Maternal anatomy and physiology 1
Maternal biomechanics 22
Melasma 17
Membrane, premature rupture of 120
Menarche 9, 129
　age of 32
Menopause, early 30
Menstrual cycle 10
　fertile days of 11, 11*f*
　phases of 9
Menstruation 9, 129
　cessation of 28
Mental
　retardation 33
　status 35
Mid-chest expansion 110
Moderate intensity resistance exercise 123

Molar pregnancy 129
　choriocarcinoma 30
Montgomery's tubercles 29, 129
Morning sickness 28
Mucous membrane 117
Mucus plug, expulsion of 120
Multigravida 129
Multipara 129
Muscle 40
　and fat 12, 47
　core abdominal 84
　exercises, abdominal 99
　stretched in pregnancy, tightening of 85
　testing 39
　twitching 129
　weakness 123
Myomas 30

N

Naegele's formula 38
National Immunization Schedule for pregnant woman 32*t*
Nausea 12, 28, 30, 119
Neck flexors 40
Nipples
　cracked 98
　sore 98
Nulligravida 129
Nullipara 129
Nutrition 34

O

Obstetric pelvis 3
Obturator internus 19
Oligohydramnios 47
Oliguria 119, 129
Opening up hip rotators 101, 102*f*
Oral contraceptives 30
Ovarian cycle 10
　phases of 9
Over birth ball 80*f*
Ovulation 8
　hormonal control of 8
Ovulatory phase 11
Oxford scale, modified 40

P

Pain 72
  abdominal 46
  chest 122
  control, mechanism of 75
  epigastric 119
  in epidural region 94
  perineal 88
Palmar erythema 17
Palmer's sign 28
Past obstetric history, record sheet of 32*t*
Pawlik's grip 36, 37*f*
Pectorals 39
Pelvic
  alignment 40
  cavity 2*f*, 3
  clock 100, 100*f*
  congestion 30
  diaphragm 17, 19
  examination 35
  floor awareness, training and strengthening 100
  floor during pregnancy and parturition 19
  floor exercise 50
    training 100
  floor muscle 17, 40, 50, 84, 98
    assessment 40
    exercises 50, 88, 112
    relaxation of 102*f*
    strength measurement, modified oxford grading for 40*t*
    testing 40
  floor relaxation 101
  girdle pain 64
  grip 36, 37*f*
  inlet 3
  lymph nodes 6
  movements, training of 100
  organs, blood supply of 3, 5*f*
  outlet 3
  rolling 112
  rotations 61
  shape 3
  tilt 93
    posterior 93*f*, 111
  tumors 30
Pelvis
  changes in 23
  female 4*f*, 4*t*
  lymphatic drainage of 6
  major 2
  minor 2
  nerve supply of 6
  pain, posterior 64
Perineal dysfunction 88
Perineal tear 82
  classification 39*t*
Peristalsis 30
Physical exercise, continuation of 85
Physiotherapy
  antenatal 42, 48, 54, 61
  management guidelines 85, 86*t*
Pigmentation 16
Pilates 123
Piriformis 19
Pituitary gland 16
Placenta 12, 47
  expulsion of 71
  praevia 130
Placental insufficiency 122
Placental separation 71
Plasma volume 13, 18
Plasminogen activator inhibitor 18
Platelet 13
  count 18
Pollakiuria 28, 130
Polycystic ovary syndrome 37, 130
Polyhydramnios 119, 122
  acute 119
  chronic 120
Polyuria 130
Postnatal assessment 38
Postnatal physiotherapy 84
Postnatal problems, long-term 98
Postoperative physiotherapy management 109
Postovulatory follicle 9
Postural changes during pregnancy 24*f*
Posture 25
  and comfort positions 57
  awareness 51
Pranayama 123
Pre-eclampsia 118, 122, 126, 130
  severe 119

Index

Pregnancy 22, 23, 42
  coagulation in 13
  common medical problems in 117
  diagnosis of 28
  duration of 37
  ectopic 128
  fibrinolysis in 13
  first trimester of 48
  mask of 127
  medical termination of 31
  multiple 33
  normal 25
  physiological
    anemia of 13
    changes during 11, 18t
  second trimester of 54
  signs of 29, 30t
  test
    home 29
    positive result of 30
  third trimester of 61
Premenstrual changes 30
Preovulatory follicle 9
Presumptive signs 30
Preterm labor 126
Primigravida 130
Primipara 130
Principal blood changes during pregnancy 13t
Progesterone 9
Protein
  C 18
  S 18
Proteinuria 19, 118, 119, 130
Pubococcygeus 19
Puborectalis 19, 20
Pubovaginalis 19
  muscles 20
Pudendal nerve 6, 17, 19
Puerperium 130
Pulsed electromagnetic energy 90

Q

Quadratus lumborum 39
Quadruped position 51
Quick contractions 101, 103

R

Radiographic study 30
Rectus
  abdominis muscle 90
  femoris 39
Red blood cell 12, 13, 18
  volume 12
Relaxation 54, 72
Renal system 15, 19
Reproductive cycle, female 8
Reproductive hormones, female 9t
Respiratory changes 18
Respiratory distress syndrome 122
Respiratory symptoms 66
Respiratory system 14
Rhinitis 34
Rhomboids 39
Rigor 46
Rocking chair 77f
Rocking, rhythmic motion 77
Routine antenatal care 45

S

Sacral nerve roots 19
Sacral plexus 6
Sacral promontory 130
Sacroiliac joint 24
  pain 64
    causes of 64
Savasana 54
  modified 62
Schizophrenia 31
Semisitting in bed 76
Semisitting position 76f, 81, 81f
Serratus anterior 40
Shoulder 51
  elevators of 39
  external rotators 40
  girdle 25
Side-lying position 59, 59f, 76f, 81, 81f
Single fetus, total weight gain for 12t, 47t
Sitting 87
  posture 57, 58f, 76f
Skin 16
Sleeping positions 59

Slow dancing 77*f*
Soft chairs, avoid sitting on 113
Sonography 29
Specific muscles
    strengthening of 88*t*
    stretching of 88*t*
Sphincter
    urethrae 19
    urethrovaginalis 19
Spider naevi 17
Spine, changes in 23
Squats, modified 56
Stair climbing 78*f*
Standing pelvic tilt 53, 53*f*
Standing posture 51, 57*f*
Stationary bicycling 49
Straddle chair 79*f*
Strength training 123
Strengthening 88
Stress 30
    incontinence 98
Stretching 88
    exercises 51
Striae gravidarum 17, 130
Stroke volume 18, 66
Superficial perineal layer 17
Superficial vein thrombosis 97
Supine lying
    during pregnancy, effect of 65
    posture 59*f*
Sway on ball 77*f*
Swimming 49, 123
Symphysis pubis 24
    pain 95

T

Tachycardia 118
Tadasana 54, 61, 62
Tailor stretching 78*f*
Tetanus toxoid 32
Thoracic area, curvature of 24*f*
Thoracic kyphosis 25
Thoracic pain 94
Three quarters lying posture 59, 59*f*
Thyroid 16
Thyroxine binding globulin 16
Tidal volume 18

Total blood volume 18
Total lung capacity 19
Toxemia 126
Transcutaneous electrical nerve
    stimulation 74, 110
    during labor, benefits of 75
    machine 75
Transversus perinei superficialis 17
Trapezius
    mid and lower fibers of 40
    upper fibers of 39
Trikonasana 61
True pelvis 2*f*, 3
    parts of 3*f*
Trunk curls 99, 113, 113*f*
Trunk rotation 53
Tuberculosis 39
Tumors 30
Tupler technique 93

U

Ujjayi pranayama 54
Ultrasound 89
    examination 30
Umbilical grip 36
Upper chest expansion 110
Ureter 130
Urinary frequency 30
Urinary incontinence 120
Urine 85
Urogenital system, female 2*f*
Uterine
    contraction 36, 130
    cycle 8
    involution 72
    signs 28
    souffle 130
Uterus 12, 47
    distended hard 120
    extra blood flow to 12
    size 85
    symphysio fundal height of 47

V

Vagina, leakage of fluid from 46
Vaginal examination 29
Valsalva maneuver 63

Varicose veins 96
Veerasana 54, 61
Vertebral bodies 23
Vigorous exercise 30
Visual changes 46
Visual disturbances 119
Visual imagery 72
Vomiting 12, 28, 30, 119
    excess 46

W

Waddling gait 23, 25, 26
Walking 49
Warm
    baths 89
    sitz bath 89

Water birth 125
    benefits of 125
    contraindications for 126
    risks of 126
Weight gain 25
    during pregnancy 12
    maternal 46
Weight loss 85
White blood cell 18
Wound support 110

X

Xiphisternum 17

Y

Yoga 54, 61, 62, 123
    and pilates, modified 123

EU GSPR Authorised Reprsentative
Logos Europe, 9 rue Nicolas Poussin
1700, La Rochelle, France
Phone: +33 (0) 6 67 93 73 78
E-mail: contact@logoseurope.eu

www.ingramcontent.com/pod-product-compliance
Ingram Content Group UK Ltd.
Pitfield, Milton Keynes, MK11 3LW, UK
UKHW021831140426
5217IPUK00021B/1386